CALM & CONFIDENT
IN THE
DENTAL CHAIR

CALM & CONFIDENT
IN THE
DENTAL CHAIR

A WORKBOOK TO HELP
EASE ADULT ANXIETY

MELIORS SIMMS

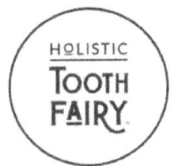

About the Author

Meliors Simms, aka the Holistic Tooth Fairy, is a natural oral health coach who helps people all over the world to avoid unnecessary dental procedures and have better experiences with the necessary ones.

After a diverse career (from policy research to craft arts) and a lifetime of terrible teeth, she turned around her own chronic dental issues by developing a uniquely holistic approach to oral health through independent research and experimentation. Today she shares the Holistic Tooth Fairy Way, a surprising toolkit of Alt Oral (Alternative Oral Health) self-help strategies, in personalised video coaching, online resources and books.

Meliors' empathetic approach to empowering fearful dental patients draws on her own history of overcoming extreme dental anxiety, as well as strategies developed through coaching hundreds of clients to get the dental care they need.

Meliors is the author of *The Secret Lives of Teeth: Understanding emotional influences on oral health,* a comprehensive guide to metaphysical healing for teeth and gums.

Table of Contents

Foreword
by Jessica Gordon DDS

Over my 14-year career working as a dental practitioner in public hospitals, private practices, and community clinics, the most common phrase I hear from patients is, "I really don't want to be here. No offense, but I hate the dentist."

On behalf of the dental profession, I apologize that this sentiment is at the forefront of so many patients' minds, even before a straightforward check-up. Anxiety about receiving dental treatment is not something for patients to be ashamed of. Rather, it's a challenge that can be addressed by both the patient and their dental clinician.

When we graduate as dental clinicians, the privilege of delivering healthcare should go hand in hand with providing emotional and spiritual support. A compassionate and empathetic chairside manner should be a lot more common in our profession than what I call 'conveyor belt dentistry'.

Throughout my dental career in New Zealand, the United Kingdom, and Uganda, I have always prioritized the patient's experience. This has included studying psychology, lighting calming scented candles and working alongside my therapy dog (Max, who is particularly popular with children). I always schedule patients' appointments to last a little longer than I think is required, to allow time for compassion and connection as well as the treatment they need.

I am acutely aware of the way people feel about coming to the dentist and my hope is that each visit with me can gradually help to ease their dental anxiety. The dentists I have worked with over the years have taught me that the best clinicians also have the best chairside manner.

However, there's also a lot that dental patients can do to prepare mentally and physically for a more positive experience. In this valuable self-help book for anxious dental patients, Meliors provides tools for a range of anxiety-inducing issues from practical advice for managing bleeding and techniques for jaw relaxation, to choosing the right dentist and communicating with your dentist effectively.

Meliors not only has a wealth of knowledge about holistic approaches to diseases of the teeth and the soft tissue, but her expertise in managing dental anxiety has me in awe. This book has shown me how I can step up my chairside game for the good of my patients. I hope more of my dental colleagues are willing to learn to do the same.

Whether you are a patient who hates going to the dentist, or a clinician who hears your patients say, "I don't want to be here", this book is for you.

Jessica Gordon, DDS

Disclaimer

The suggestions in this book have been collected and curated from a variety of sources and tested by me and my clients in our real lives as ambivalent dental patients.

When choosing to try the activities and practices in this book, you should consider your personal circumstances to decide whether they are appropriate for you. You need to take responsibility for your own health and wellbeing.

I am not a dental or psychological professional and I am not offering dental or psychological advice. I try to provide valuable information, but I cannot be responsible for the use you make of that information.

The suggested activities and practices in this book are for educational and informational purposes only, to help you make better health decisions in conjunction with your regular treating practitioners. In choosing to follow any of these suggestions, you are taking responsibility for your own actions. Please use common sense before following any of the suggestions.

GET READY WITH DENTAL PREP

The lowest point in my lifelong dance with dental fear happened under general anaesthetic, so I don't remember it. But I still shudder when recalling the shame of being woken to learn the procedure was stopped because I was crying and thrashing around while unconscious.

That's when I realised that the dental profession had run out of ways to handle my extreme dental anxiety and it was past time to find my own solutions.

These days I'm a natural oral health coach who helps people to avoid dental procedures when possible and to overcome their dental ambivalence when needed. But for a long time, I suffered the consequences of having terrible teeth despite my dedicated compliance with mainstream advice.

I don't have professional expertise in dentistry, unless you count the subjective ten thousand hours I've spent being worked on (or worked over) in the dental chair. I exaggerate, of course, but I really have spent a lot of time getting fillings, root canals, crowns, and extractions.

Some of those hours in dental offices ranged from pleasant to tolerable. Most of my dentists have been kind and competent.

But over the first 45 years of my life, I endured too much dental work that was unnecessary or badly done (or both), that was often painful, and was usually expensive. Eventually, those negative experiences accumulated to the point that I started having panic attacks at the dentist.

At first, I could mask my state of terror in anticipation of appointments so that I appeared only normally apprehensive. But eventually, I couldn't help but cry quietly in the waiting room. Then the tears followed me into the dental chair to the extent that I would moan and twitch uncontrollably, despite my best efforts to keep still and quiet.

My lovely dentist had been dealing with my escalating distress over a couple of years when he recommended my sixth root canal. He suggested putting me under with general anesthetic to ensure I would stay still through the drilling. I agreed because it sounded like sleeping through it could be the solution I needed.

because it sounded like sleeping through the procedure could be the solution to my dental distress.

I expected to wake up once the procedure was complete. To my surprise, when I came to consciousness in the dental chair, I found out that the root canal had barely begun and my partially drilled tooth was packed with temporary filling. I was (kindly) told to sort myself out before coming back to finish the procedure.

That afternoon, I contacted a hypnotherapist specializing in dental fears and phobias. A handful of hypnotherapy sessions proved to be the turning point in my relationship with dentistry. A few weeks later, I went back and completed the root canal procedure without interruption. The next time I had a dental crisis, I was able to avoid a seventh root canal by researching alternative solutions and that's how I became immersed in the wild and often wacky world of alternative oral health.

Ultimately, the best remedies for my dental anxiety turned out to be following effective nutritional guidelines, jaw exercises and optimized hygiene protocols to have strong, healthy resilient teeth and gums. I much prefer going to the dentist when I don't have to get drilled.

Nonetheless, one legacy of my earlier decades was a mouthful of less-than-perfect restorations, which sometimes still need to be repaired or replaced. Over the last decade I've had plenty of opportunities to develop an extensive toolkit of ideas for patients to improve any dental experience.

Together with my coaching clients, I've experimented to refine, improve and expand my personal dental prep toolkit into a robust, multifaceted series of activities to prepare for appointments, and practices to use in the dental office.

Tailor your own toolkit

This book gathers together the most universally useful dental prep activities from my coaching toolkit. It includes all kinds of techniques that have helped me, and/or my clients, to avoid or minimize feelings of anxiety, confusion or helplessness at the dentist's.

In the following pages, I will guide you through many of the same practices that I share with my one-on-one clients, including:

- insightful journal prompts for you to gain more clarity about your dental priorities,

- simple activities to help you prepare physically and psychologically,

- practical tips for staying calm in the dental chair, and

- guided visualizations and meditative practices*

Some of the recommendations might not be relevant or helpful for you or your current situation. You certainly don't have to do all twenty-five activities before your next dental appointment!

*If you would like to listen to my voice guiding you through some of these meditations, download bonus content mp3 audio recordings at :

https://holistictoothfairy.com/calm-confident-bonus

DENTAL AMBIVALENCE

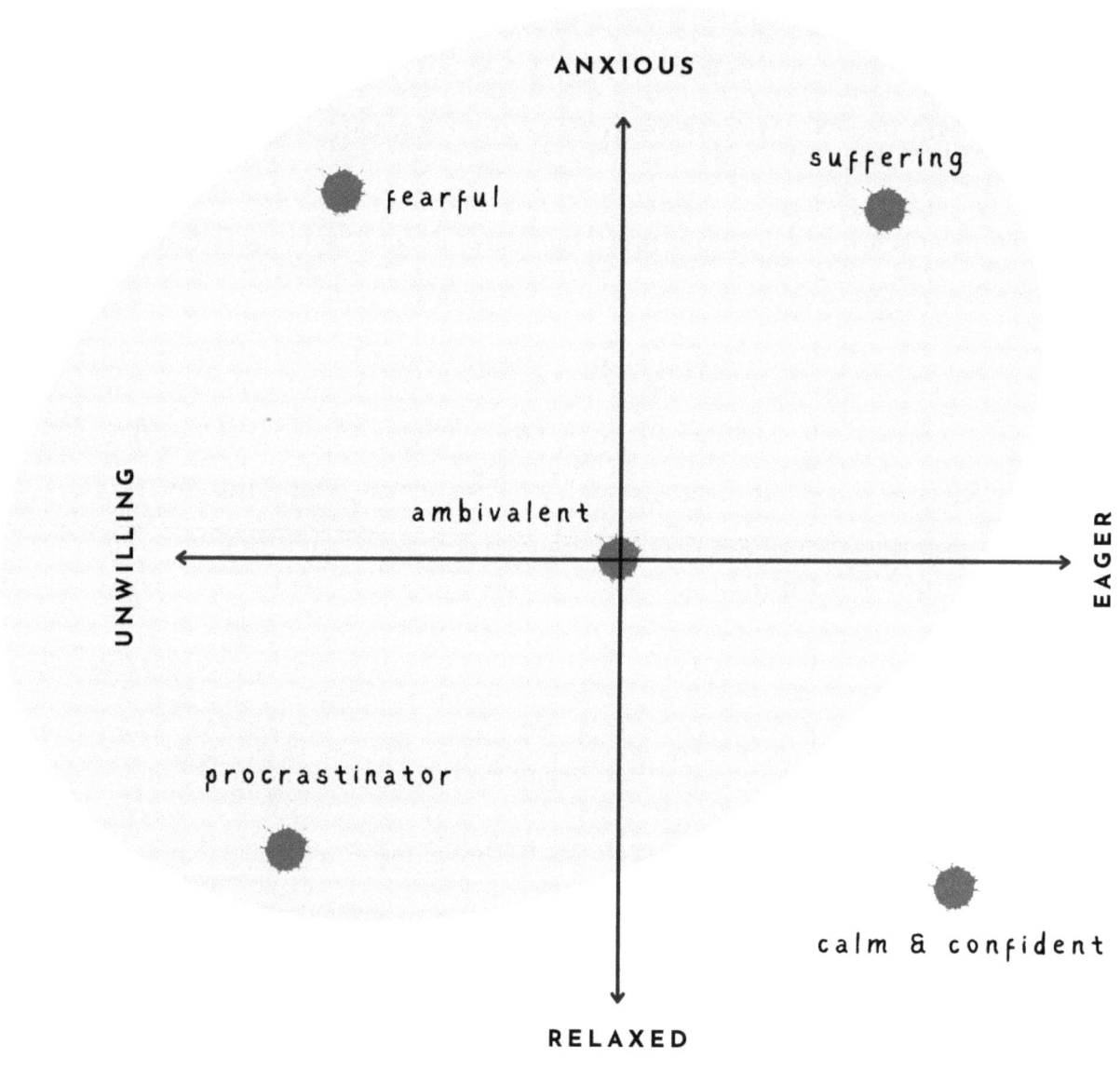

The Dental Ambivalence Scale

This book is intended to help anyone who places themselves in the gray oval to the top and left of the Dental Ambivalence Scale. Working through the activities in this book should help you to shift your feelings about the dentist toward the open space of the lower right quadrant.

To help you decide which activities will be most useful for you, first think about where you sit on the Dental Ambivalence Scale on the opposite page.

Identify where you sit on the scale right now and make a mark with today's date.

You can repeat this exercise again after you have done some or all of the activities, just before or after you go to your next dental appointment, and when you prepare for future dental appointments.

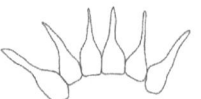

Visualize yourself at the dentist

Imagine walking through the dentist's door

feeling calm and confident.

Picture yourself explaining clearly

what you do and don't want

and your dental team responding

with respect, patience, and support.

See yourself lying back comfortably

as the dentist gets to work inside your mouth.

The time passes easily

and before you know it,

the appointment is over.

Imagine getting up out of the chair,

feeling pleased with the experience

and at peace with the outcome.

This idealistic vision is possible for you, even if you've never felt that way before and aren't sure it's realistic; and especially if your anxiety is getting in the way of your best interests.

It's not irrational to feel afraid of the dentist. Lying on your back with someone else's fingers in your mouth is an inherently helpless feeling. It's hard to think logically and make good decisions in that position, or immediately afterward. You may feel like you don't have any control, so if you are someone who only feels safe when you are in control, it's scary.

It's true: you **are** giving up some control in that moment when you 'open wide' in the dental chair. You **are** vulnerable to the dentist's intentions and level of skill. Dental procedures **may** be uncomfortable.

But you can have a lot more control than you might think. Your past dental experiences don't have to define your future. You can establish trust with your dentist before you lie back in the chair. There are ways you can minimize or at least cope with pain or discomfort.

As you develop more confidence and calm, your dentist becomes more competent*. Dentists pick up on your fears and it may subconsciously compromise the quality of care they provide and the converse is true too.

You can use this book to move yourself down and right on the Dental Ambivalence Scale. Maybe you won't get all the way to 'eager and willing' at your next visit, but I believe that you **can** dramatically improve your immediate experience.

---

*Wherever you see italics centered like this,
it's a passage to be used as guided visualization or meditation.*

When you see left-justified italics like this, it's passage to be used as journal prompts.

When you see a box like this, it's a place for you to pause and make some notes.

This book is designed for **doing,** not just reading. If you revisit the activities in this book during the week or two before each future dental appointment, you will gradually grow more calm and confident But only if you **do** the work in this book.

You'll need to engage with at least some of the activities: the ones that address your particular flavor of dental anxiety. The next activity will help you plot the best course from your current state of dental ambivalence to the state you want to be in for your next dental appointment

---

* Hamezelou, Jessica, Dentists can smell your fear – and it may put your teeth at risk, New Scientist, 25 May 2018

1 Choose Your Own Adventure

In this activity you can organize your dental prep plans for between now and your next appointment. Create a plan that suits the time you have available and the aspects of the dental visit that are most uncomfortable for you.

This activity will be especially helpful if you:

- like knowing exactly what you should do and when
- benefit from the external accountability of a checklist
- are dealing with many competing demands on your attention.

If you prefer to work through the activities spontaneously at your own pace, you can skip this chapter.

Think back over your whole life and all the challenges you have already overcome.

What kind of practices have worked for you to handle anxiety or stress in other contexts?

Are there transferable tactics or strategies you can apply to your dental ambivalence?

Include them in your personalized plans.

The suggestions on the following pages are organized primarily by what particular challenges you may face with going to the dentist.

Within those categories the suggestions are organized according to the time you have available between now and your next dental appointment, depending on whether you:

- open this book for the first time on the same day as your dental visit,
- start working through the activities in the week or two leading up to an appointment, or
- are looking for motivation to book your first dental appointment in a long time.

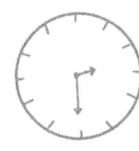

If you only have one day or less to prepare, choose from the suggestions under 'when you have hours'.

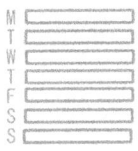

If you have 2-13 days to prepare, add in suggestions from 'when you have days'.

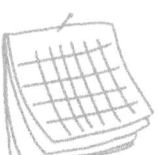

If you have more than two weeks to prepare, add in suggestions from 'when you have weeks'.

Bookmark, highlight or underline the activities you want to do and check them off as you complete each one.

Anxious about physical discomfort/pain

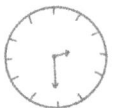 When you have hours   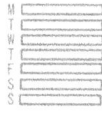 When you have days   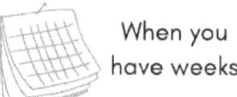 When you have weeks

5. Cradle your jaw

6. Massage your jaw

7. Stretch your jaw

13. Dental calm

14. Focus on breathing

15. Prepare your mind

20. Hand signals

21. Before you say goodbye

23. Your dental story

24. Forgiving the past

Overwhelmed with sensory sensitivi-

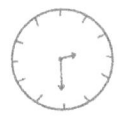 When you have hours    When you have days   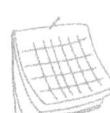 When you have weeks

13. Dental calm

14. Focus on breathing

15. Prepare your mind

16. Prepare your ears and eyes

20. Hand signals

2. Managing emotions

10. Exploring ambiva-lence

11. Intentions and boundaries

21. Before you say goodbye

23. Your dental story

24. Forgiving the past

Emo-

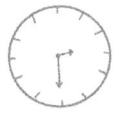 When you have hours

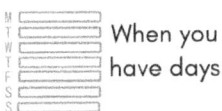 When you have days

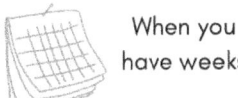 When you have weeks

21. Dental calm

14. Focus on breathing

15. Prepare your mind

16. Prepare your ears and eyes

20. Hand signals

10. Exploring ambivalence

11. Intentions and boundaries

19. Empowering body language

21. Before you say goodbye

22. Confident dental decisions

23. Your dental story

24. Forgiving the past

Difficult dental history

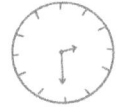 When you have hours

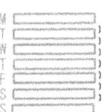 When you have days

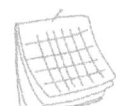 When you have weeks

21. Dental calm

14. Focus on breathing

15. Prepare your mind

19. Empowering body language

2. Managing emotions

10. Exploring ambivalence

11. Intentions and boundaries

18. Empathetic communication

21. Before you say goodbye

22. Confident dental decisions

23. Your dental story

24. Forgiving the past

Avoiding the dentist

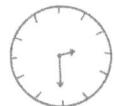 When you have hours

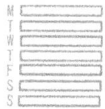 When you have days

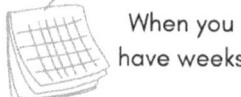 When you have weeks

14. Focus on breathing

19. Empowering body language

21. Before you say goodbye

17. Talk about teeth and gums

10. Exploring ambivalence

11. Intentions and boundaries

3. Making dental appointment

12. Changing or choosing your dentist

22. Confident dental decisions

23. Your dental story

24. Forgiving the past

Unclear about your dental needs

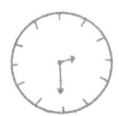 When you have hours

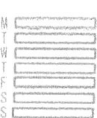 When you have days

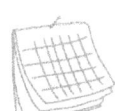 When you have weeks

17. Talk about teeth and gums

2. Managing emotions

10. Exploring ambivalence

11. Intentions and boundaries

22. Confident dental decisions

Anxious about communicating

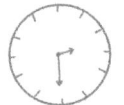 When you have hours

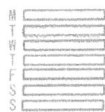 When you have days

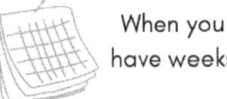 When you have weeks

17. Talk about teeth and gums

19. Empowering body language

20. Hand signals

10. Exploring ambivalence

11. Intentions and boundaries

18. Empathetic communication

21. Before you say goodbye

22. Confident dental decisions

Worried about gagging

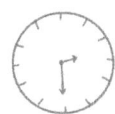 When you have hours

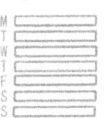 When you have days

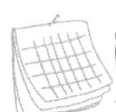 When you have weeks

5. Cradle your jaw

6. Massage your jaw

7. Stretch your jaw

9. Prepare not to gag

20. Hand signals

13. Dental calm

15. Prepare your mind

10. Exploring ambivalence

11. Intentions and boundaries

14. Focus on breathing

16. Prepare your ears

18. Empathetic communication

21. Before you say goodbye

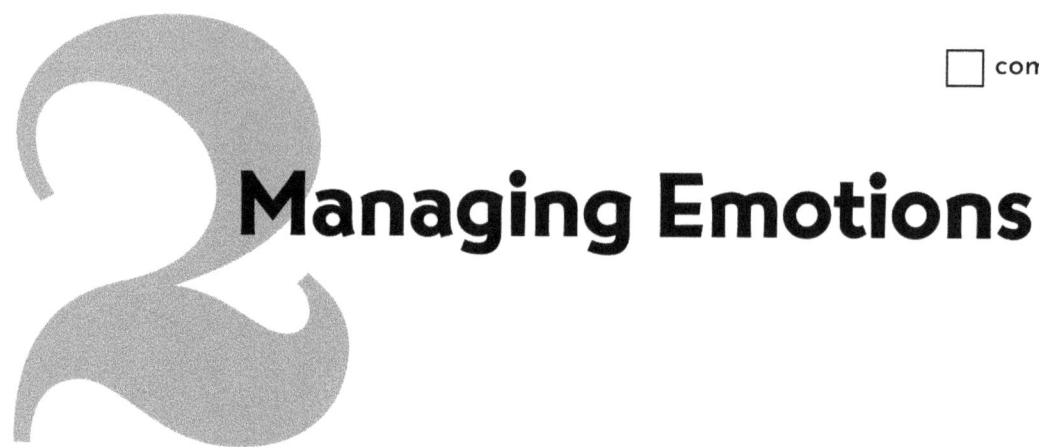

☐ completed

2 Managing Emotions

Some activities in this book may bring up uncomfortable memories of going to the dentist, if that's been part of your story.

You may feel some strong feelings that you had been hoping to avoid. Be mindful of when and where you do these exercises, to allow yourself time to release emotions and integrate your insights.

If needed, seek support from a professional or trusted friend as you work through the activities.

Whether you are doing this book alone, or with external support, make sure you feed, water, and rest your body before attempting any of the more introspective activities.

This activity will be especially helpful if you:

- have strong emotional reactions when thinking about the dentist
- are doing any of the visualizations or journaling activities (e.g. activities 11, 12, 22, 23)

If you have strong feelings while doing any of the activities try any of these suggestions to manage your emotions:

- Slow mindful breathing (see Activity 14).
- Havening technique (see Activity 61).
- Emotional Freedom Technique aka EFT aka tapping (see Activity 22).
- Move your body to release tension e.g. dance, walk, run, jump.
- Cry, scream, shake or laugh as needed.

Reorientation ritual

This is a short practice that you can use after any of the other activities in this book to minimize the risk of becoming stuck in difficult emotions that might get stirred up by thinking about your dental appointment (or dental history).

It will help you move more easily onto the next thing you want to do in your day (or to fall asleep afterward if you do activities at night). You can also use it on leaving the dentist's, or any time you think it might be helpful.

Take a deep breath.

Wriggle your fingers and toes.

Stretch your arms

and change your posture.

Look around and notice that

you are not at the dentist's right now.

Focus your eyes on something that makes you feel safe.

Do you need to have a sip of water,

go for a walk, or take a nap?

Be gentle with yourself as you address your own ambivalence, resistance or fear of the dentist. This is important work and it may not be easy or straightforward. Treat this scared part of yourself with kindness and compassion.

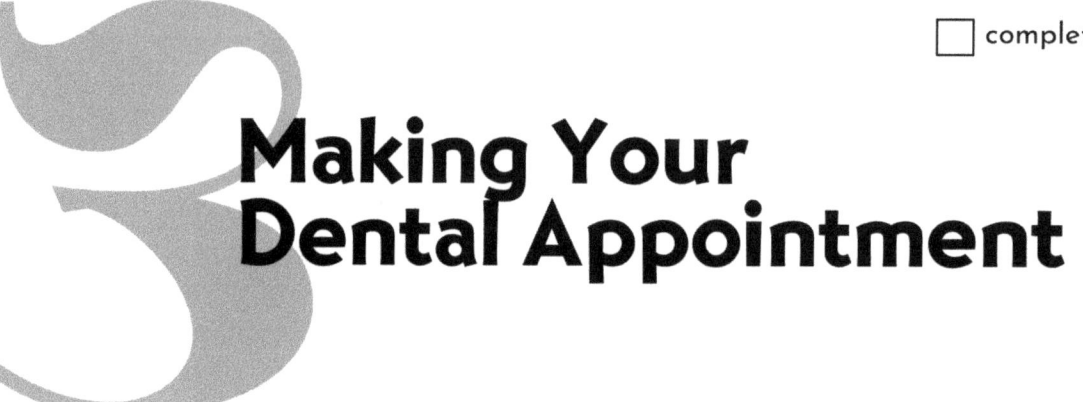

☐ completed

3 Making Your Dental Appointment

This activity addresses some of the practical considerations that may get in the way of scheduling a dental appointment.

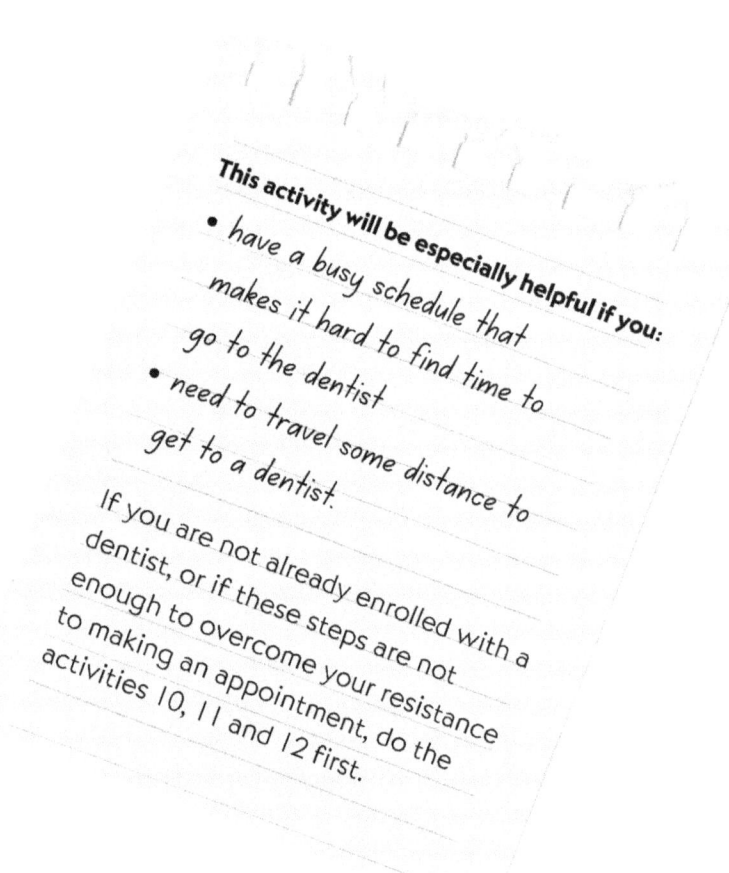

This activity will be especially helpful if you:

- have a busy schedule that makes it hard to find time to go to the dentist
- need to travel some distance to get to a dentist.

If you are not already enrolled with a dentist, or if these steps are not enough to overcome your resistance to making an appointment, do the activities 10, 11 and 12 first.

Steps to booking an appointment

Once you know the booking procedure, it will be easier to take action to schedule your appointment, either right now or the next time the office is open.

Find out whether the dentist's practice prefers to take bookings online or by telephone, or both.
If both are available, would you prefer to book online or by telephone?

Find out how far in advance you need to book. Many dental practices can get booked up weeks in advance. Look on their website or make a quick call to find out what their wait time is.

Some people find it easier to overcome unwillingness, ambivalence, or procrastination by booking a dental appointment weeks (or months) in advance. You can always reschedule closer to the date.

Or, if you are still feeling unwilling to act, continue working through the rest of the activities in this book until you feel ready to schedule an appointment.

Is it an emergency?

If your symptoms include any of the following, you should see a dentist or doctor immediately:

- fever
- difficulty breathing
- difficulty opening your mouth completely
- unbearable pain that can't be eased
- a new wisdom tooth in the lower jaw at the same time as pain and a bad taste in your mouth.

Describe your symptoms when requesting an urgent appointment.

If you having a dental crisis and need urgent care, you can ask to get on your dentist's cancellation list. They may recommend another dental practice or an emergency dental service. Some hospital emergency departments provide a dental service, but this should be your last resort.

Other symptoms which mean that you should see your regular dentist as soon as possible include:

- pain that gets worse at night
- a tooth which is sensitive to hot, cold or tapping
- a lump with pus on your gum
- painfully swollen gums with a bad taste in your mouth
- loose teeth or loose gums
- any sore, lesion or ulcer in your mouth that lasts more than two weeks.

Timing your appointment

If your dental appointment is not an emergency, think about what date, day of the week, or time of day will make it easier for you to arrive at the dental office feeling calm and confident.

Do you need to arrange time off work?

Will you need to return to work after the appointment?

What if you have a numb mouth or feel shaky after the appointment?

Can you schedule a dental visit so that you can go home to rest afterwards?

Consider traffic and parking, or public transport timetables, at different times of day.

Will you be under pressure to collect your children from school or daycare afterwards? Can you ask someone else to pick them up on that day?

Eating before and after

If you have are going to have a numb mouth, make sure you nourish yourself well before the appointment in case you're not be able to eat for a few hours afterwards. Consider organizing some soft or liquid food ready for later in the day if needed.

4 Things To Bring

This activity is a reminder to note down things that you want or need to bring with you to the dentist, based either on your past experiences, or as suggested by the following activities. This page is bookmarked so you can find it again easily while working through the rest of the book, and so that you can refer to it on the evening before, or morning of your appointment day.

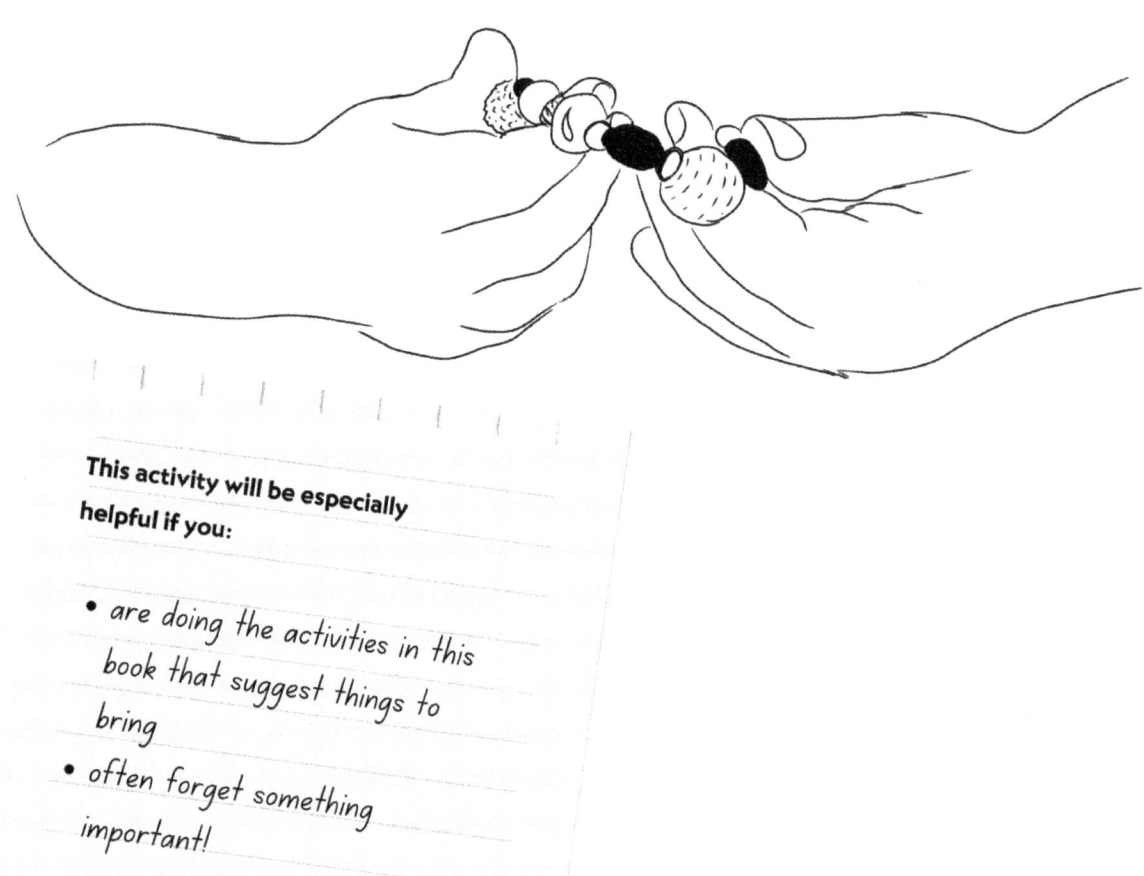

This activity will be especially helpful if you:

• are doing the activities in this book that suggest things to bring

• often forget something important!

THINGS TO BRING

THING	WANT	WHERE	READY
YOUR NOTES (THIS BOOK?)			
YOUR DENTAL RECORDS			
MUSIC (PLAYLIST ON DEVICE)			
EARBUDS OR NOISE CANCELLING HEADPHONES			
SLEEP MASK			
READING GLASSES			
SOMETHING SMALL TO HOLD ONTO			
SALTWATER RINSE			

Which of the things that you could bring, do you want to bring?

Where are the things you want to bring?
Do you need to borrow or buy anything?

Check the READY column when that item is organized
and packed up to take along on the day.

PREPARE YOUR MOUTH

In this section, the activities focus on preparing your mouth and jaw for a dental appointment. The next three activities will help you to feel more physically comfortable opening your mouth wide in the dentist's chair.

I suggest starting to prepare your mouth at least a week before your next dental appointment. I've put these activities near the beginning of the book to allow you plenty of time to repeat them as often as possible (e.g., once a day) in the lead-up.

However, even a single session of 'open wide' preparation in the hours before an appointment will help a lot.

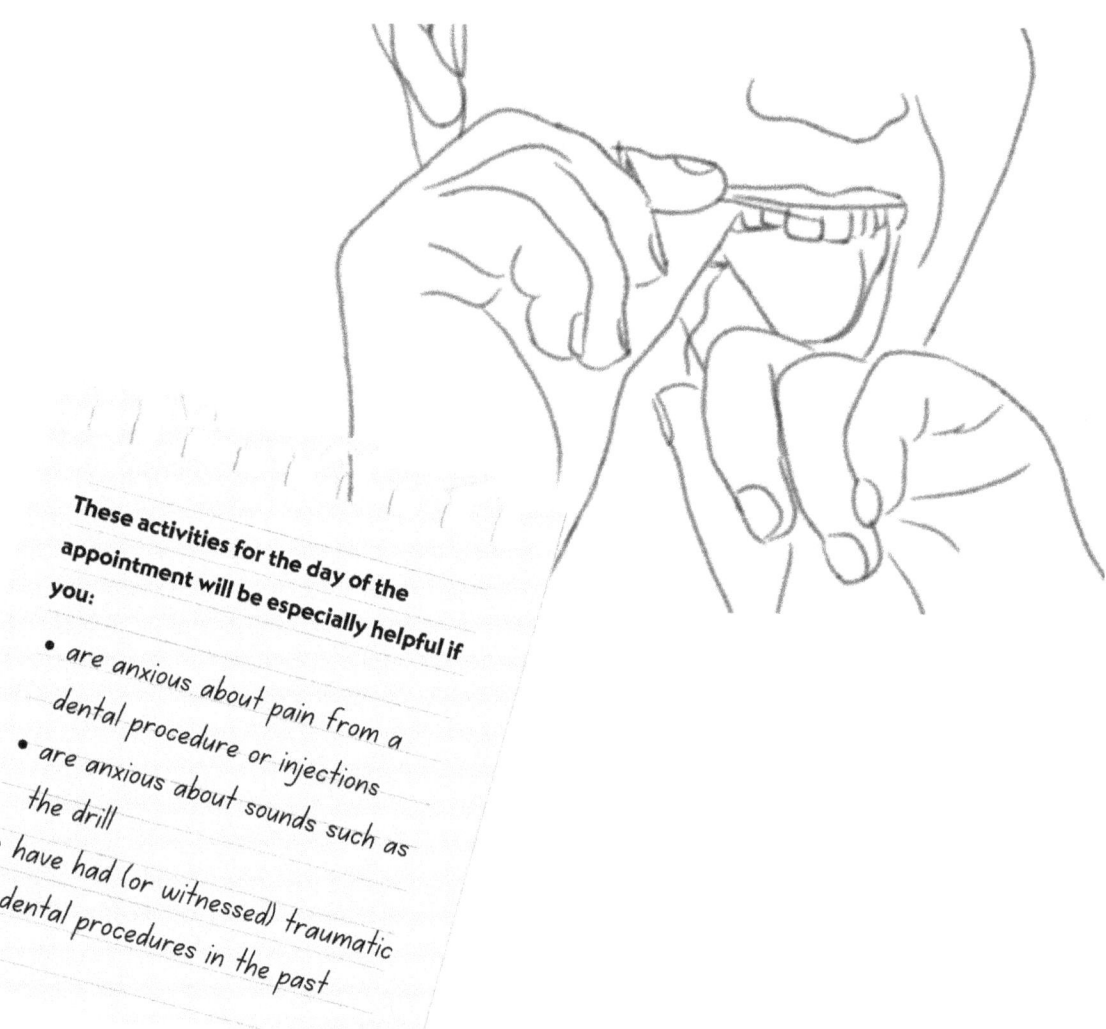

These activities for the day of the appointment will be especially helpful if you:

- are anxious about pain from a dental procedure or injections
- are anxious about sounds such as the drill
- have had (or witnessed) traumatic dental procedures in the past

Open wide

Most dental visits require you to open your mouth very wide for some amount of time. This could be at least 15 minutes for a check-up, thirty minutes for a cleaning or a simple restoration, or even longer for a complicated procedure like multiple fillings, a root canal or an extraction. You'll have to open the widest for work on your wisdom teeth or top molars.

Just like other parts of your body, your jaw can become more flexible with regular stretching. However, if you have trouble opening your mouth wide without your jaw clicking or seizing up, if you have TMJ* disorder or another serious jaw condition, please use your best judgment about how you practice the jaw stretch (Activity 7).

The open wide prep sequence includes three activities. You can do any of them separately, but they are most effective when you do all three in this order:

1. Cradle your jaw

2. Massage your jaw

3. Stretch your jaw

I encourage you to do the whole sequence before bedtime because it may also help stop you from clenching or grinding your teeth in your sleep.

It's just as helpful for dental prep to do it first thing in the morning (maybe even while you are still in bed) or to link it with your toothbrushing habit to help you remember. (Tip: the massage feels great to do while you are applying moisturizer to your face). Even a single session of 'open wide' prep in the hours before an appointment will help a lot.

For a long procedure, ask if your dentist or hygienist has a bite block available to help you keep your mouth open for extended periods of time without discomfort.

---

* Temporomandibular joint (the hinge between upper and lower jaws)

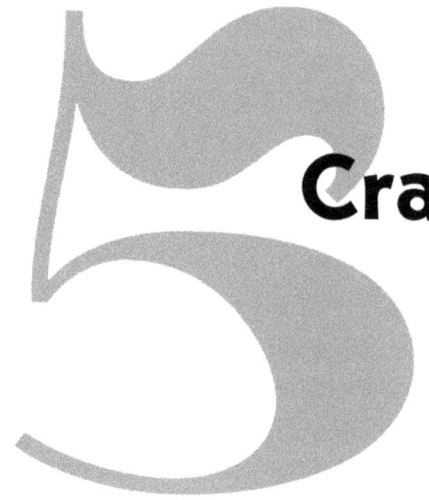

☐ completed

Cradle Your Jaw

Start by sending your jaw some loving compassion.

Rub your hands together to get warmth in your palms.
Cup your jaw in your hands.

With your chin resting on the heels of your palms and your fingers rest-
ing in front of your ears, take a slow deep breath in through your nose,
and slow breath out through your nose.

Keep up this slow steady breathing through the whole sequence.

Now imagine that you are holding in your cupped hands
a tiny baby animal: maybe the cutest little kitten or puppy
you have ever seen in your life.

Imagine its soft, furry, floppy little body resting so lightly in your hands.
See how it's gazing up at you
with bright, trusting, curious eyes.

Let yourself feel that feeling of, 'Oh! You are so cute!'
Let that feeling rise up through your body and flow through your hands
into your jaw.

Spend a few moments basking in that feeling of tender compassion,

then start the Massage Your Jaw activity on the next page.

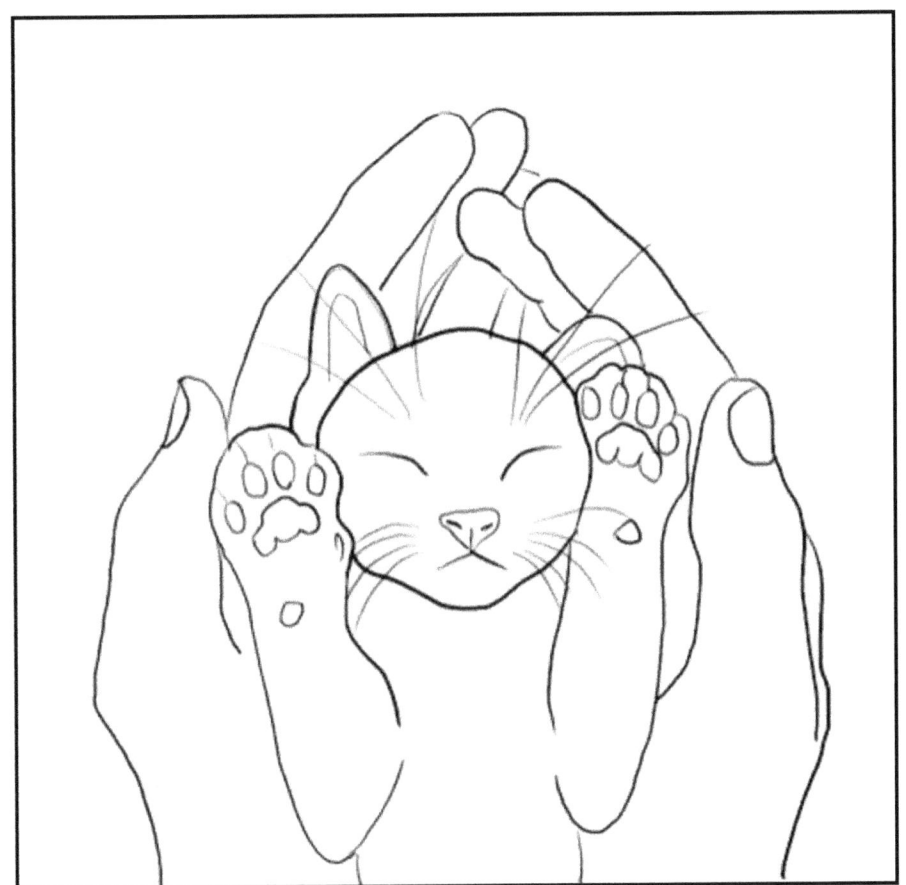

1. Cradle your jaw lovingly on the way into the dental office or in the waiting room.
2. Cradle your jaw lovingly after the appointment.
3. Cradle your jaw lovingly before or after any of the activities in the rest of this book (you'll find an extended version included in Activity 10).

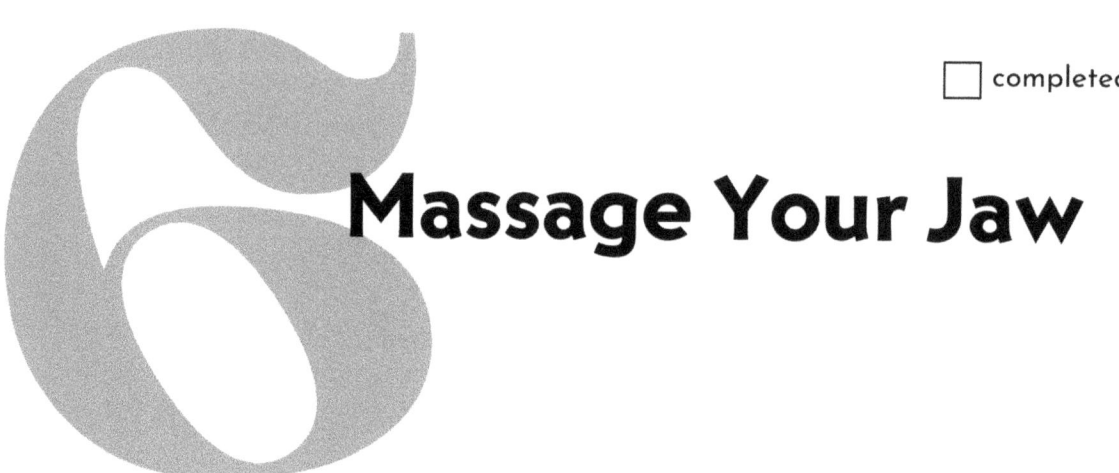

6 Massage Your Jaw

Massage your jaw following these steps, going very slowly, mindfully and gently while paying attention to your breath. Try to stay with each step for at least a minute.

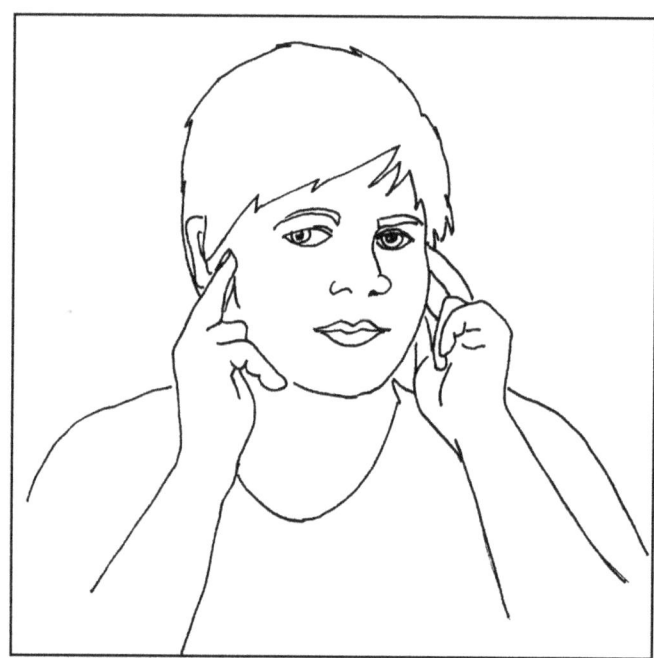

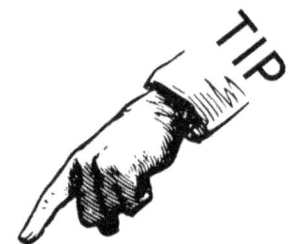

Breathe through your nose and keep your chin tucked so your neck stays straight throughout this exercise.

1. Massage the TMJ joint which is the hinge between your upper and lower jaws. You can feel it as a hollow indent just in front of your ears. Press your fingers in and around the hollow.

2. Massage along your upper jaw by moving your fingertips in slow circles as though you are massaging your top gums through your cheeks. When your fingers meet under your nose, go back slowly along the upper jaw again.

3. Massage along your lower jaw by moving your fingertips in slow circles as though you are massaging your lower gums through your cheeks. When your fingers meet under your bottom lip, massage in slow circles back along the lower jaw again.

4. Massage underneath your jaw, at the top of your throat with the tips of your thumbs. Start at the corner of your lower jawbone under each ear. When your fingers meet under your chin, massage circles back along under your jaw again.

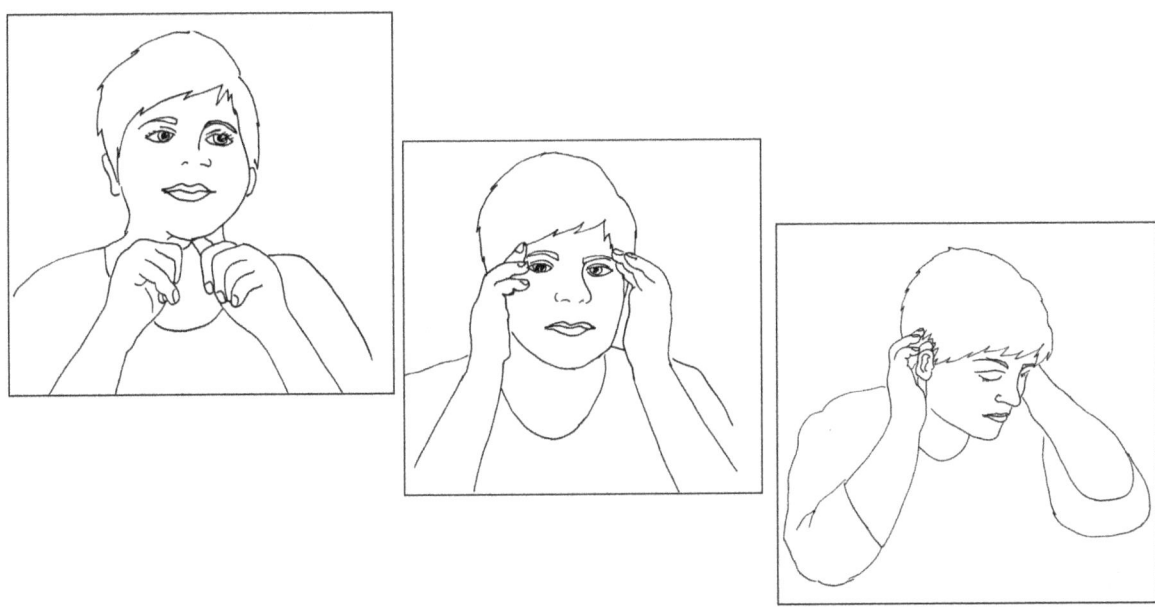

5. Lightly massage small circles all the way around your eye sockets with your fingertips a couple of times. Stroke your fingertips from the center of your forehead over your temples to your TMJ. Stroke your fingertips from the bridge of your nose across your cheekbones to your TMJ.

6. Massage firm circles over and down behind your ears. Massage circles along your neck at the base of the skull until your fingers meet at the occipital notch where the spine enters the skull. Extend the massage to your scalp, neck, and shoulders as desired.

When you are finished massaging your jaw, move onto the next activity to stretch your jaw muscles in preparation for comfortably opening wide at the dentist's.

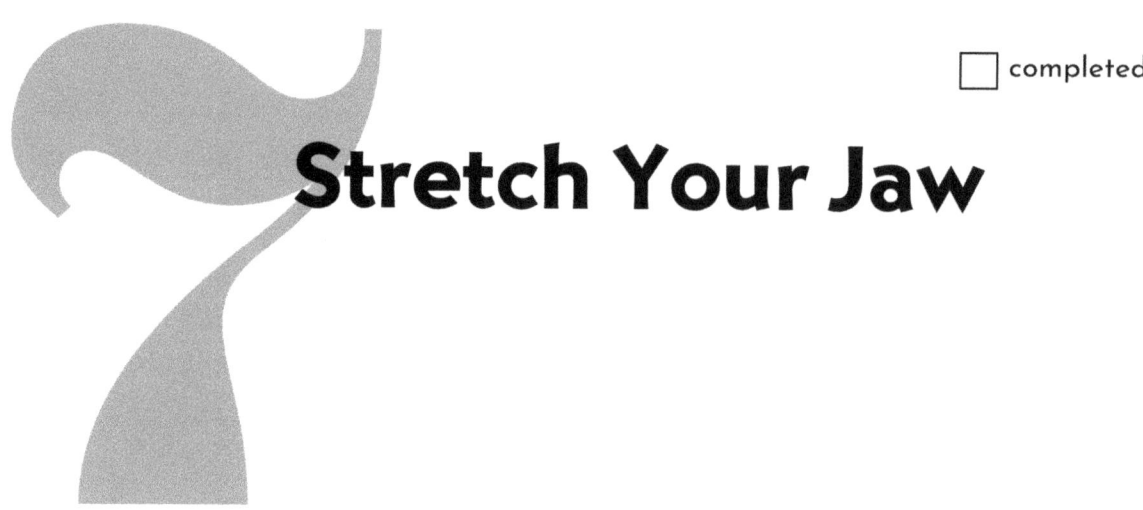

Stretch Your Jaw

Now that your jaw is nicely relaxed, stretch your mouth wide open into a giant noisy fake yawn.

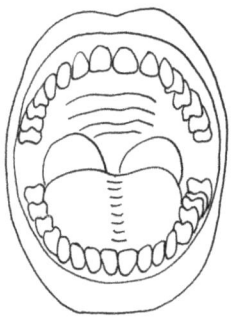

Stretch as wide as is comfortable for you (note: it's not a competition to open the widest).

Making a noise while you stretch helps to relax your muscles so you can open wider and more easily (and allow emotional release).

If you have a clicky jaw, stretch to just before the point you click, without clicking.

You'll probably find it easier to open wider after two or three days of practice.

Say WOW like you are faking a big yawn.

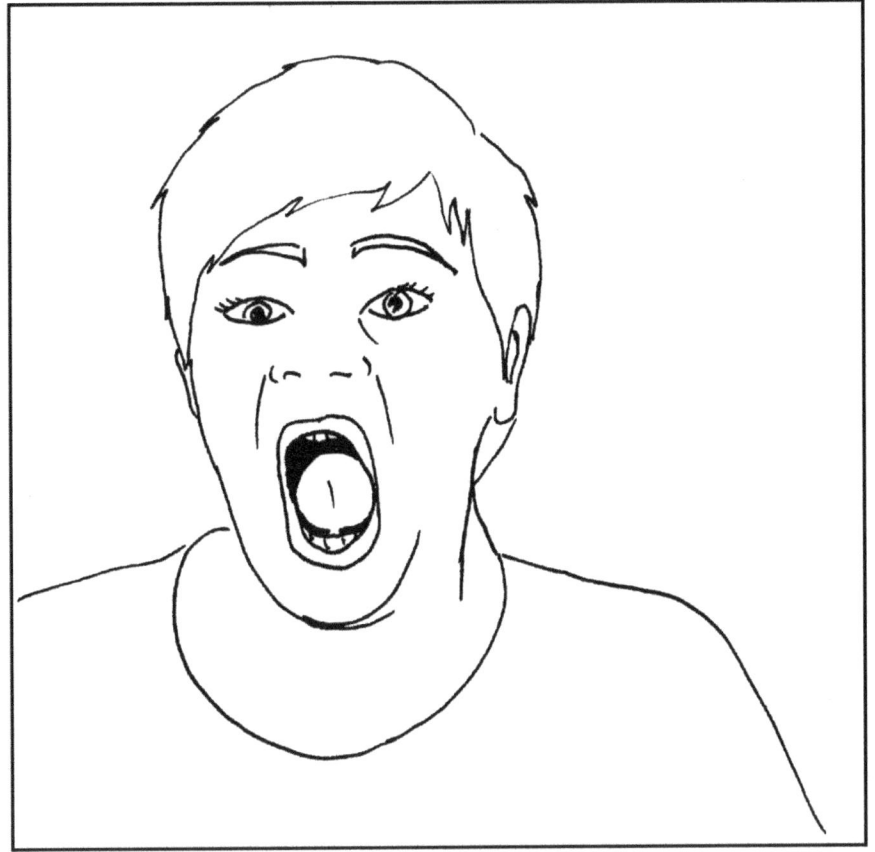

Repeat these fake yawns or WOW stretches 10 times in a row.

(Real yawns count).

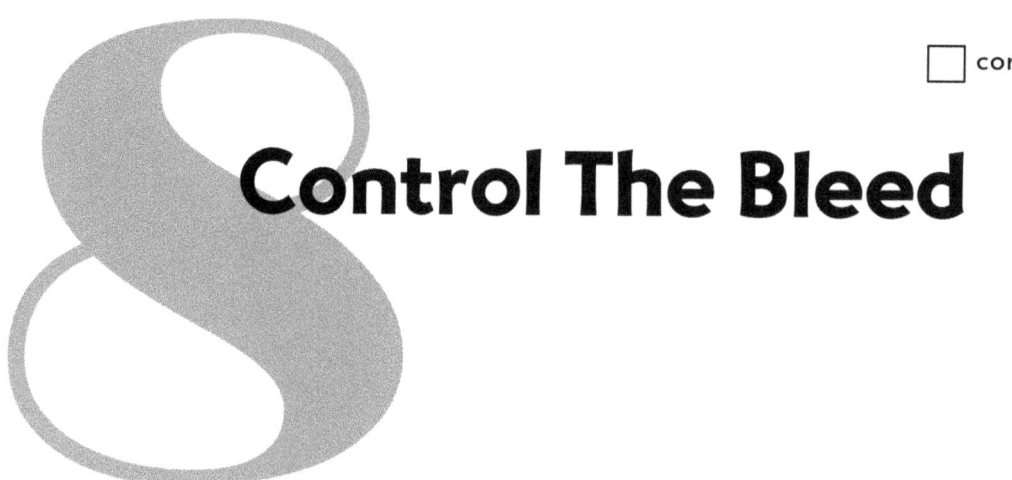

□ completed

8 Control The Bleed

In this activity, the focus is on building up resilience in your gingiva (gum tissue) to minimize the amount that you bleed with the hygienist.

It might seem counterintuitive, but if **occasional** flossing makes you bleed, there's a good chance that **frequent** flossing will reduce the amount you bleed during a dental cleaning. Flossing or other gumline and intraoral cleaning techniques help reduce the bacterial load on those parts of your gingiva, making your gum tissue stronger and more resilient.

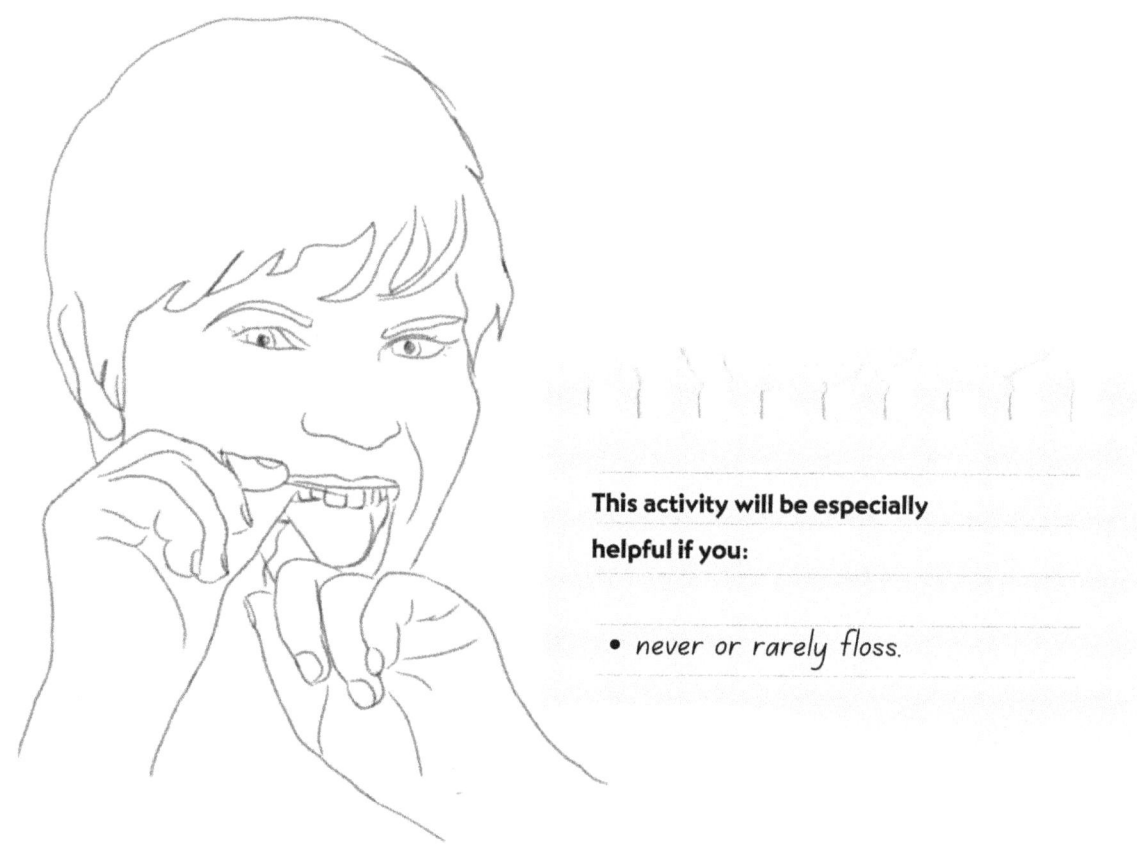

This activity will be especially helpful if you:

• *never or rarely floss.*

Flossing Technique

Start with a fresh piece of string or tape floss about the length of your forearm.

Wrap most of it around one index finger and wrap the short end around your other index finger.

Gently ease it in between two teeth, with a back-and-forth motion, being careful not to slam it into your gum.

Pull the floss into a firm loop around one of the teeth, so that it touches the base of the tooth at the level of the gum.

Rub the floss gently and mindfully in a shimmying motion (like drying your back by pulling the ends of a towel) three or four times.

Loosen the loop, then lift it slightly away from the gum before you switch the direction of the loop to wrap it around the adjacent tooth.

Rub the floss gently and mindfully back and forth around the other tooth three or four times .

Pull the floss out from between your teeth and wind it onto your finger to expose a fresh, clean stretch of floss.

Repeat between all your teeth. Don't forget the back of the last tooth in each quadrant of your mouth.

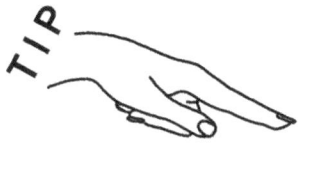

Avoid using floss picks (short pieces of floss attached to a handle) as these can distribute bacteria around your mouth and damage your gums.

Choose the best kind of floss for your teeth.

If you have tight crowded teeth, choose a fine, slippery floss such as silk. If even the finest, slipperiest floss is too hard to get between all your teeth, try using a water flosser (oral irrigator) or small size Piksters (intraoral brushes).

If you have more ease between your teeth, choose a thicker, more textured floss such as charcoal-infused bamboo.

Water flossers and larger Piksters can be great for widely spaced teeth as well.

Rinse after eating

Try rinsing your mouth with a saltwater solution after every time you eat. Swish in your mouth, then spit.

Saltwater solution

Dissolve one tablespoon of salt in two cups of spring water.

1. Bring your own bottle of saltwater solution to the dentist if you don't like their minty-fluoride mouthwash.
2. If you have a bad reaction to saltwater rinse, just use plain tap water to rinse after eating or experiment by rinsing with a cool herbal tea such as chamomile, sage, or peppermint.

Prepare Not To Gag

This activity may help you not to gag on a mouthful of dental equipment. Dental x-ray sensors, especially at the back of your mouth, can make some people feel like gagging. Having your mouth filled with dental impression materials to make a mold for dentures or a mouthguard is another kind of dental procedure that can cause gagging.

If your gagging sensitivity is an emotional trauma response, just using the physical and sensory tips below may not be enough. You may need to take this challenge into a therapeutic conversation or work with a trauma specialist to address the specific associations you have with gagging.

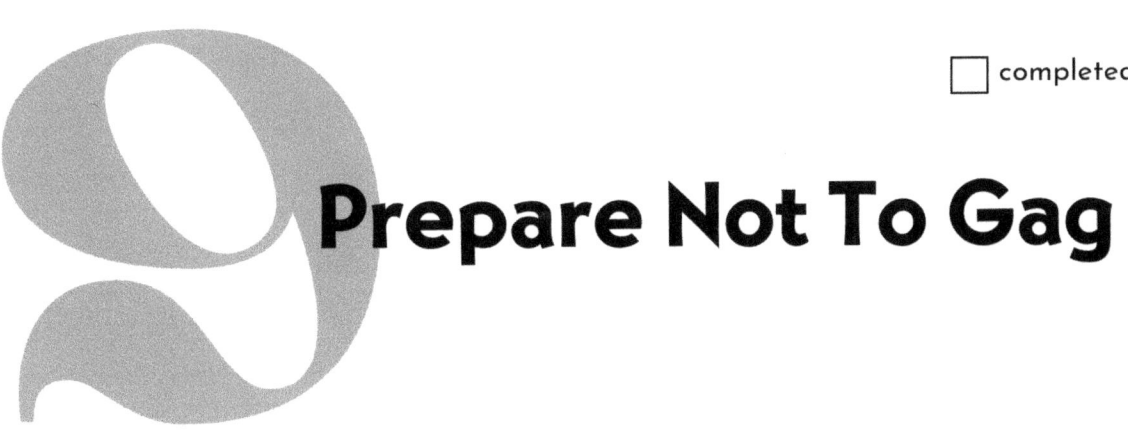

This activity will be especially helpful if you:

- have a strong gag reflex
- have trouble brushing or flossing your back teeth without gagging
- have gagged on a dentist's fingers, x-ray sensor or other equipment in the past
- expect to have an impression taken inside your mouth.

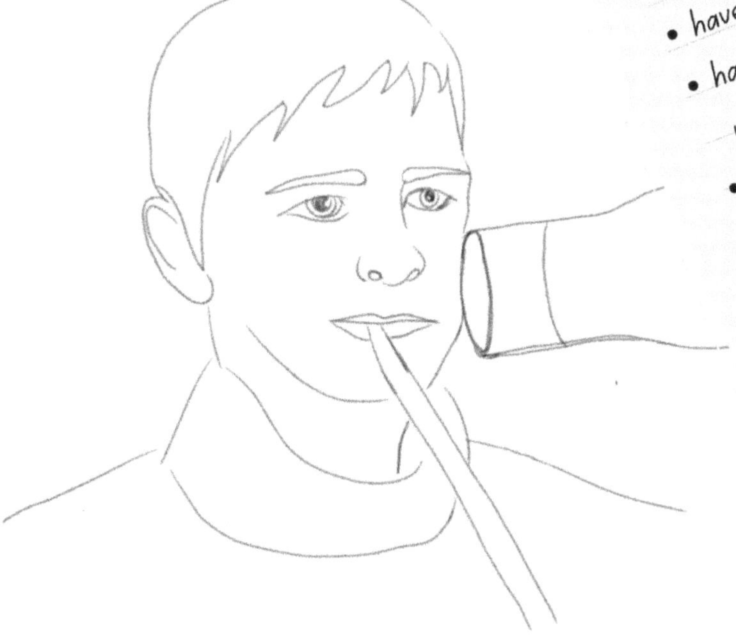

Explain to the dentist that you have a strong gag reflex, so they can be extra careful. They may even have some tips and tricks of their own for avoiding a gagging reflex.

Read through the list of tips that other people have found helpful. Write the date of your next appointment next to 1-3 tips that you can use at this time. After the appointment, make brief notes about what happened and whether each tip was successful.

NO-GAG STRATEGIES

SUGGESTION	DATE TO TRY	RESULT
SWALLOW BEFORE THE X-RAY SENSOR GOES IN YOUR MOUTH		
DON'T SWALLOW WHEN SENSOR IS IN YOUR MOUTH		
ASK IF YOU CAN FINE TUNE POSITIONING OF SENSOR		
PUT A PINCH OF SALT ON YOUR TONGUE FIRST		
TILT YOUR CHIN DOWNWARDS		
CONSCIOUSLY TRY TO RELAX YOUR TONGUE		
WRIGGLE YOUR TOES OR STROKE YOUR FINGERS TOGETHER		
HUM WITHOUT MOVING YOUR HEAD		
PRACTICE BREATHING THROUGH YOUR NOSE		
LISTEN CLOSELY TO HEADPHONES OR EARBUDS		
PLAN TO THINK ABOUT SOMETHING PLEASANT OR DISTRACTING		

UNDERSTAND YOUR AMBIVALENCE

The activities in this section will help you to prepare yourself psychologically, emotionally, and energetically for your next dental appointment.

Set aside some time to tune into the inner wisdom of your mouth. This will help you be clearer about what you need to happen, so your next dental appointment can be a more positive experience.

If you have a history of dental trauma, these activities may bring up some uncomfortable feelings for you. Please be discerning about where and when you follow these prompts. Use the *Reorientation Ritual* from Activity 2 to close the session and allow yourself enough time to reset your nervous system afterwards. Reach out for support from a trusted professional or friend if needed.

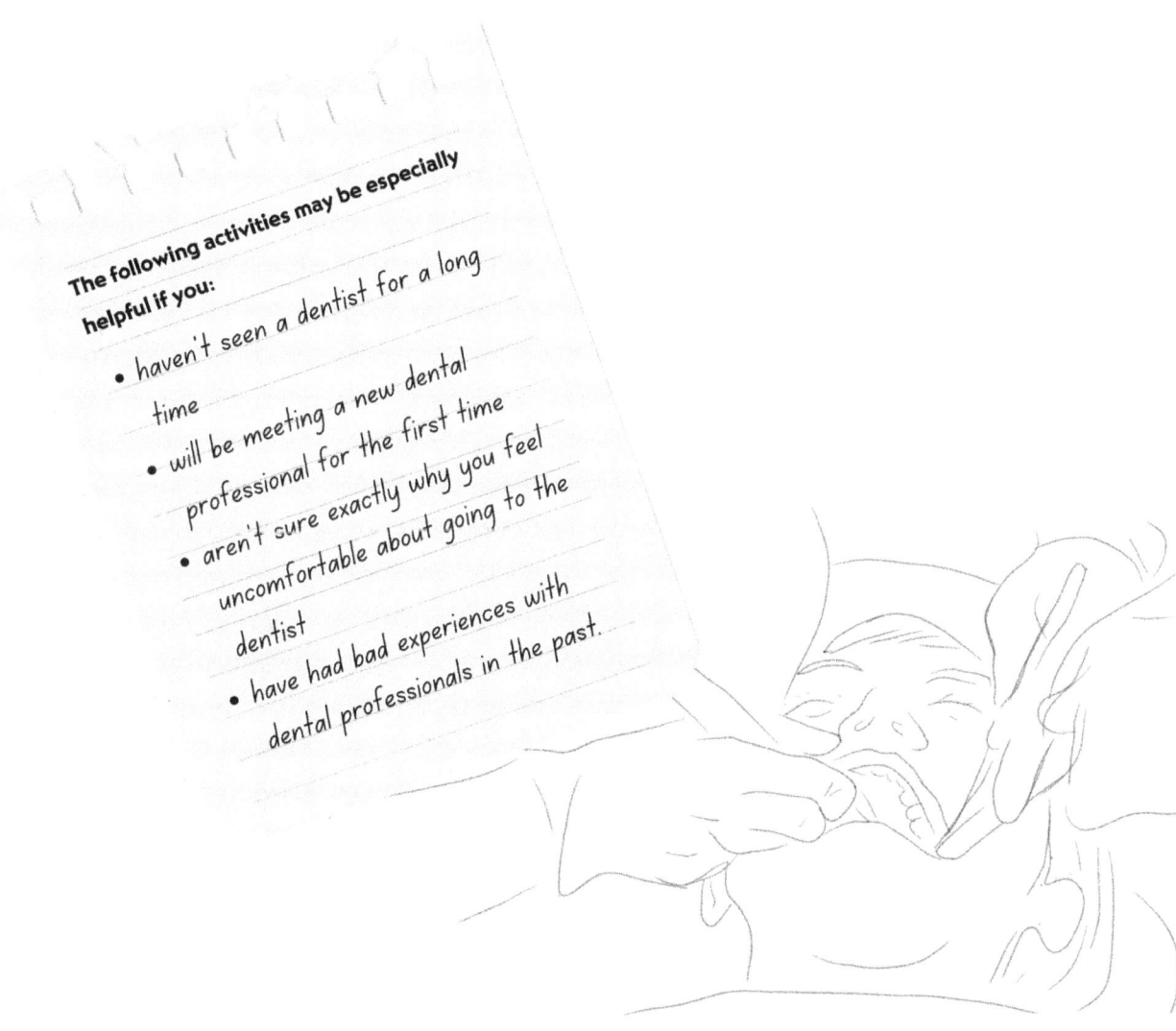

The following activities may be especially helpful if you:

- haven't seen a dentist for a long time
- will be meeting a new dental professional for the first time
- aren't sure exactly why you feel uncomfortable about going to the dentist
- have had bad experiences with dental professionals in the past.

10 Exploring Ambivalence

This introspective activity is intended to help you unpick the tangled threads of your dental ambivalence. Exploring your thoughts and feelings more deeply than usual may bring additional insights as to why you feel unwilling or anxious about the dentist. With this renewed self-knowledge, you will be able to prepare for a more positive experience and better communication at the dental office.

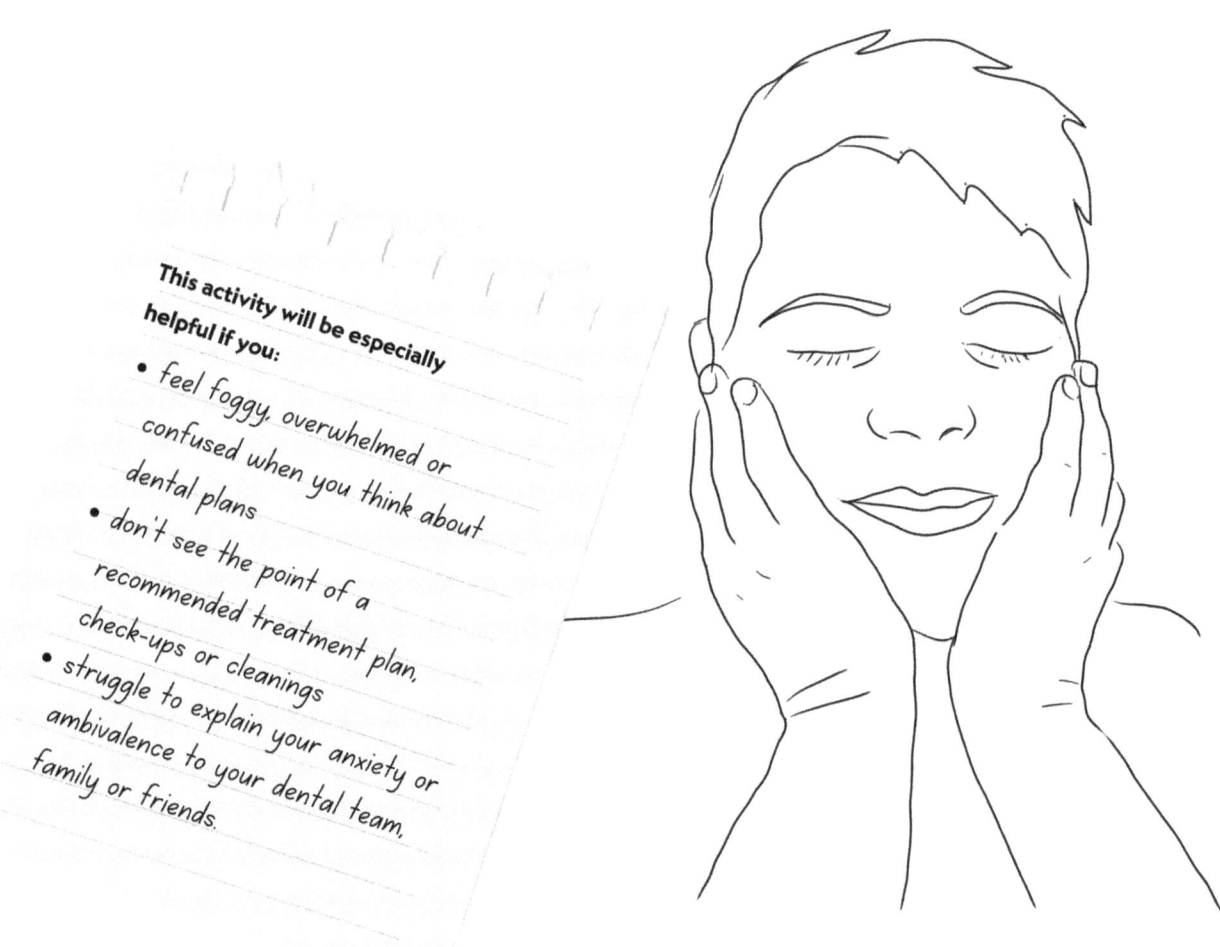

This activity will be especially helpful if you:

- feel foggy, overwhelmed or confused when you think about dental plans

- don't see the point of a recommended treatment plan, check-ups or cleanings

- struggle to explain your anxiety or ambivalence to your dental team, family or friends.

You may choose to do this activity:

- as a guided visualization,

- as journal prompts,

- alternating between meditation and journaling, or

- in a therapeutic conversation, e.g., talking it through with a professional or trusted friend.

Guided Visualization

Most people find it easiest to do a visualization meditation by listening to the words*. Download a recording in the bonus content to listen to me guide you through the meditation in my New Zealand accent (link on page 3) or this QR code.

Alternatively, you can record a more familiar accent by reading the words aloud yourself (or ask someone else to read them) into a voice recorder to play back later.

Journaling

If you prefer journaling over meditation, you can read the words of this activity silently to yourself as you follow the directions and engage your imagination as you write.

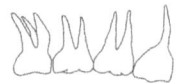

Begin with sending your mouth some love.

Rub your hands together to get warmth in your palms.

Then cup your jaw in your hands

so your chin is cradled between your palms

and your fingers are resting in front of your ears.

Take a slow deep breath in through your nose,

and slowly breathe out through your nose.

Keep up this slow steady breathing through the whole visualization.

Now imagine that you are holding in your cupped hands

a tiny baby animal: perhaps

the cutest little kitten or puppy you have ever seen in your life.

Imagine its soft, furry, floppy little body resting so lightly in your hands.

See how it's gazing up at you with bright, trusting, curious eyes.

Let yourself feel that feeling of, oh! you are so cute!

Let that feeling rise up through your body

and flow through your hands into your jaw.

Let your whole mouth marinate in the feelings of tender delight,

unconditional affection, compassion, and love

that are often easiest to access with baby animals.

Now, put your attention inside your mouth.

Imagine telling your teeth, gums and jaw

about your next dental visit and why it's needed.

As you use words or images to describe what's planned,

notice any sensations or emotions and where you feel them...

in your mouth or elsewhere in your body.

Offer tender compassion to the parts that are reacting to your plans.

Make a note of these observations.

Ask your mouth for its support in getting necessary dental care.

Notice what and where you feel sensations or emotions

in response to making this request of your mouth.

Ask your teeth, gums and jaw what they need

in order to be willing and able to accept dental care.

Make a note of any ideas, images, feelings or words

that come into your awareness.

What does your inner wisdom want you, or the dentist, to know?

Make a note of any ideas, images, feelings or words

that come into your awareness.

What does your body need to be physically comfortable

at your next dental visit?

For example, what do you already know

about your sensitivity to pain or sensory overload

that needs to be considered at the dentist's or hygienist's office?

What do you need the dental team to be aware of

about your sensitivity to sensory overload or pain?

Ask your mouth what your inner child needs

in order to be able to trust your dental team on the day?

Make a note of any ideas, images, feelings or words

that come into your awareness.

Consider if there could be a perceived power imbalance

between you and your dental practitioner

due to age, gender, ethnicity or some other quality

that could be exaggerated by lying back in the chair?

Scan your body for physical sensations as you explore this question.

Is there anything in your past that needs attention now

in order for you to be able to stay fully present

right through your next dental visit?

For example, have you had trauma that could get reactivated

by lying on your back under an apparent authority figure

or by having things put in your mouth?

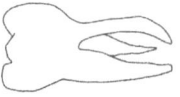

When it feels like you've spent enough time with this focus,

take a deep breath.

Wriggle your fingers.

Stretch your arms or change your posture.

Look around, notice that you are not at the dentist right now.

Focus your eyes on something that makes you feel safe.

Do you need a drink of water?

Do you need to move ?

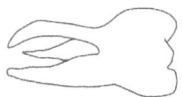

If this activity has stirred up some big feelings, please take a few minutes to remember and make note of what resources, support people and tools you have access to for working with strong emotions.

Make use of those resources to address the issues that get in the way of accessing dental care.

Take a break and then come back after a few hours or a few days to read over the insights and reflections that you noted during this activity.

Highlight or underline key points or emotionally intense phrases in your notes. Add more ideas as they come to you.

BOUNDARIES

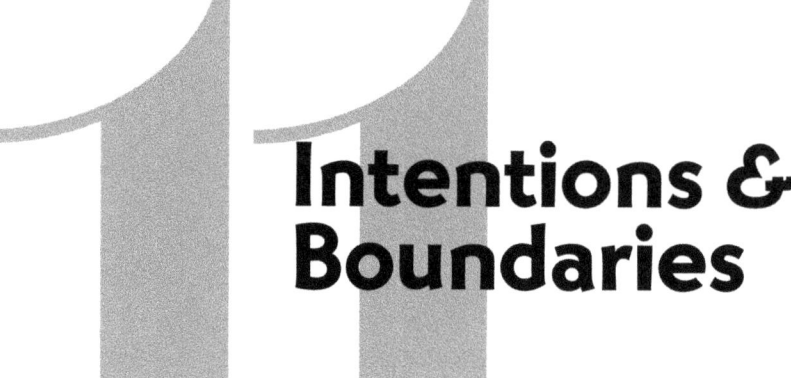

11 Intentions & Boundaries

The purpose of this activity is to help you identify what you want and don't want to happen at your upcoming dental appointment or cleaning.

Thinking through, and writing down, clear statements of your intentions and boundaries before you get to the dental office will help you be better prepared to communicate confidently and calmly with your dental team.

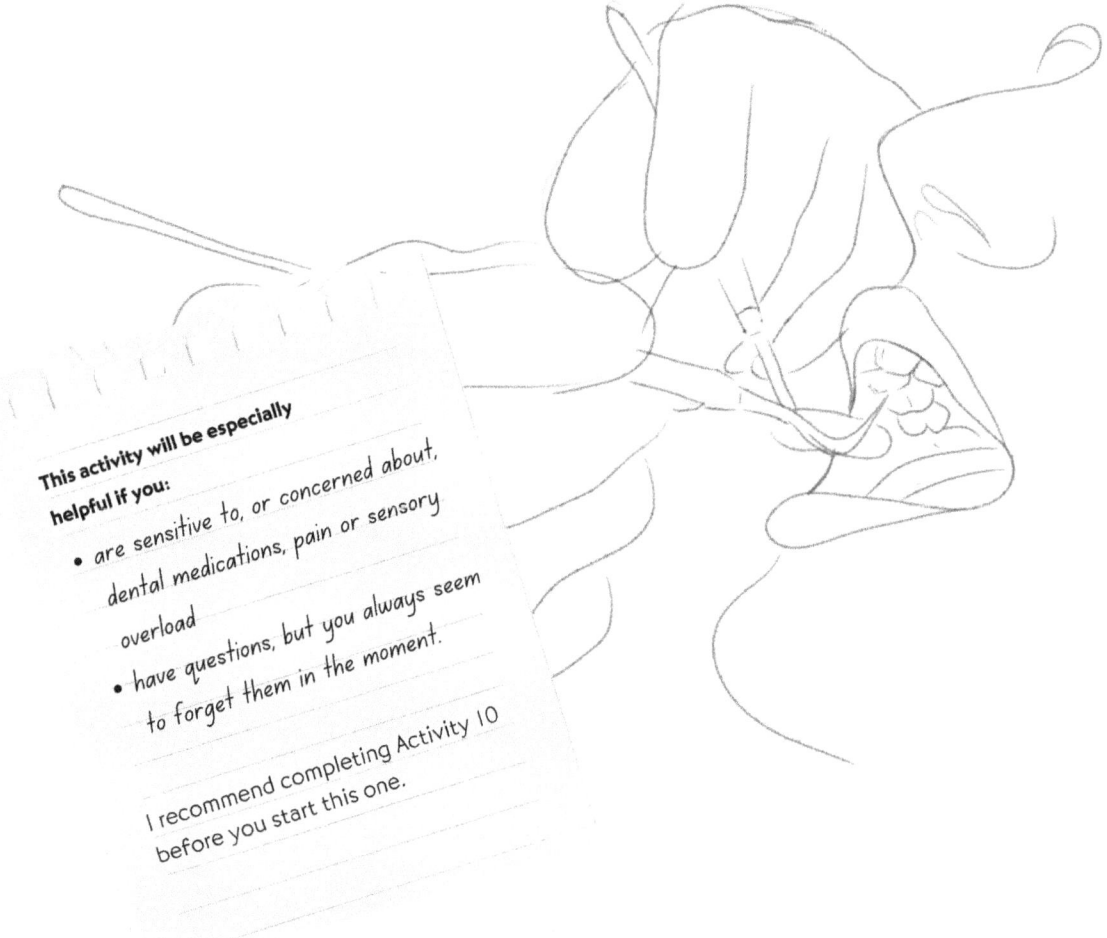

This activity will be especially helpful if you:

- are sensitive to, or concerned about, dental medications, pain or sensory overload

- have questions, but you always seem to forget them in the moment.

I recommend completing Activity 10 before you start this one.

Identifying intentions

Think about what you want to experience at the dentist's.

Are there particular medications that you want, such as local anaesthetic ?

*What do you need to be physically comfortable in the dental chair
or during a procedure?*

*What are specific questions that you want answered before any work
begins?*

Do you want the dental team to explain everything they do during the appointment? Do you want them to ask for consent before every procedure during this appointment?

Is there anything else you can think of that you definitely want to happen at your next dental visit?

Establishing Boundaries

Think about what you don't want to experience at the dentist's.

Do you have problems with any medications that you should avoid?

Are there certain materials or procedures that are a concern for you?

Would you prefer to not know what's happening during the procedure and only be given a summary once the work is done?

Do you have a budget limit for the cost or co-pay for your treatment?

Is there anything else you can think of that you don't want to happen at your next dental visit?

Add more ideas as they come to you over the next few days.

What to share

Your dental team may need to know some (but not all) of your intentions and boundaries. Make a note of what you definitely want or need them to know.

For example, your dentist or hygienist should be informed about:

- sensitivity to pain or sensory overload
- fear of needles or other specific dental tools or practices
- any allergies or concerns with dental materials or medicines
- wanting to bring a support person into the dental surgery with you
- what recent symptoms you've observed with your teeth and gums
- any new lumps or lesions either inside or outside of your mouth (including your entire head and neck)
- what questions you want answered.

Summarize what to tell the dental team here.

Advance actions

Review your notes and consider which of your intentions and boundaries the dental team might need to know **before** you arrive at your appointment. Schedule a time to send the dental practice an email or to make a phone call.

Are there other items from your intentions and boundaries notes that you need to act on before your appointment? Transfer those items to your calendar or daily to do list to so you don't forget.

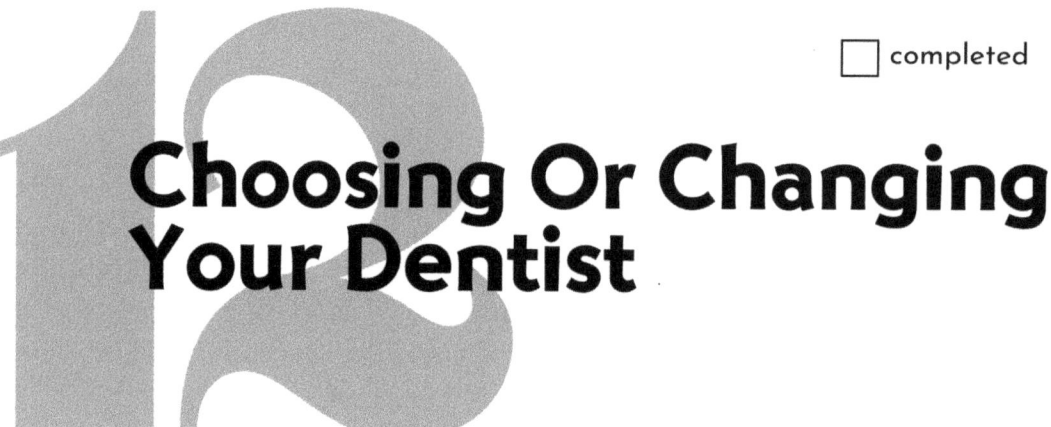

Choosing Or Changing Your Dentist

This activity offers some suggestions to help you find a new dentist or hygienist you can trust. Believing that your dental professional can be trusted; both as a clinician and a human can be a significant influence on your capacity to feel confident under their care.

I recommend doing Activity 11 *Intentions and Boundaries* first, to be clear about what matters most to you in your dental experiences.

This activity will be especially helpful if you:

- have been avoiding dental care or check ups because you aren't happy with your current, or most recent, dentist

- have moved to a new area since your last dental visit.

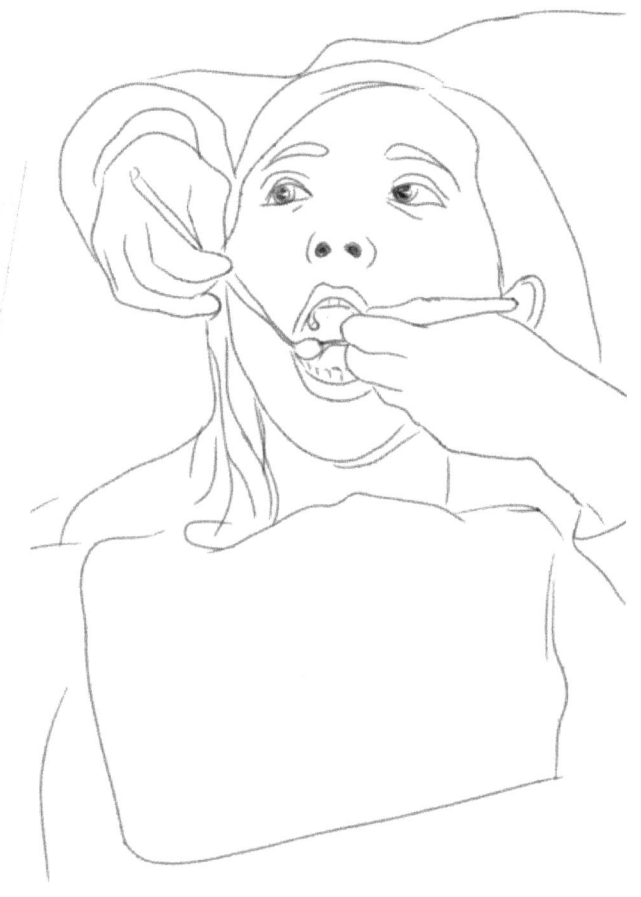

What criteria are you looking for in your next dentist?

Do you need a dentist who prioritizes being extra-gentle?
Do you need a hygienist who allows time for slow careful cleanings?
Do you need a dentist who is liberal with painkillers?
Do you need a dentist who is conservative with interventions?

Do you need a well-regarded specialist with expertise
in implants, root canals or orthodontic adjustments etc
Do you want a dentist whose practice aligns with
your holistic health values?

Do you want your dentist to be open minded
to your non-mainstream perspective?
Do you want a dentist to be respectful of your needs and preferences?
Do you want a dentist who uses, or doesn't use, particular equipment (e.g.
laser) or materials (e.g. amalgam fillings).

DENTIST

Do you need a dentist who is walking distance, driving distance or accessible by public transport from home, work or school?

Do you need a dentist whose office is easily accessible for wheelchairs or prams?

Do you need a dentist who accepts your insurance?
Do you need a dentist whose fees fit your tight budget or who won't try to persuade you into expensive cosmetic treatments?

What other factors are important for you in a dentist?

'Holistic' dentists

If your priorities include avoiding standard dental materials or procedures, you might think that you should look around for a holistic dentist. But you'd be wrong. I'm sorry to say that the term 'holistic dentist' is vague, unregulated, and virtually meaningless.

Some dentists who identify as 'holistic' (and some who appear mainstream) may practice in a way that is aligned with your holistic health values but others will not. If you are committed to finding a dentist who practices in a way that takes the whole-body system into account (i.e. avoids toxins etc.) then you are generally better off searching for terms like:
- biological dentist,
- integrated dentist,
- functional dentist, or
- bio-mimetic dentist.

Unfortunately, there aren't very many such dentists practicing anywhere in the world outside of a few big cities. You may need to travel and/or wait for months to get an appointment with one of these dentists.

Fortunately, many mainstream dentists will respect your intentions and boundaries if you state them clearly and empathetically. It **is** possible to get dental care aligned with your values in a regular dental practice when you find the right dentist and establish a positive connection.

Choosing a dentist you can work with

Start collecting a shortlist of up to three dentists who look likely to meet at least some of the criteria you identified in the first part of this activity. Search online (e.g., google 'dentist near me' or search for 'dentist' in local Facebook groups) and ask friends, colleagues and neighbors for their recommendations.

Not everyone has the same priorities for their dental care, so take the time to ask **why** your friend recommends this dentist. Some other ways to find out more about your possible future dentist include:

• reading reviews online (but bear in mind these may not be reliable)

• asking a dentist's peers or colleagues (i.e. other dentists, hygienists or receptionists)

• requesting a short phone call or interview with the dentist prior to your examination appointment, and

• reflecting on how you feel after your first contact with the dentist.

You may want to find out:

• Do other patients feel respected by the dentist?

• Is the dentist open-minded?

• Is the dentist a good listener?

• Does the dentist hear their patients' concerns and honour their requests?

• Is the dentist willing to adjust their office practices to meet special needs?

• Does the dentist always explain their decisions and gain consent before they take an action?

Although I use the term dentist throughout this activity, the same questions can apply to choosing a new dental hygienist, periodontist, orthodontist or other specialist.

Distant dentists

Many parts of the world are 'dental deserts' where there are no, or few, dentists practicing locally. If it is impossible to find a dentist nearby, or at least one you want to work with, then you may have to travel for dental treatment to the nearest big city or even further afield.

International dental tourism destinations may offer much more affordable services for major restorations (and perhaps the opportunity to vacation in a sunny, exotic place while you are having your teeth fixed). However, the quality can be extremely variable: from world class excellence to incompetent or exploitative.

If you are travelling to see a dentist, check their reviews and references, and take the time to tune into your gut feelings. I recommend completing or repeating the *Intentions and Boundaries* Activity 11 specifically in relation to a dentist you have to travel to see.

Complications from procedures performed far from home are more difficult to resolve than when things go wrong with a local dentist. The distant dentist may be unreachable once you return home. Where possible, I recommend working with a dentist with whom you can have a sustained relationship.

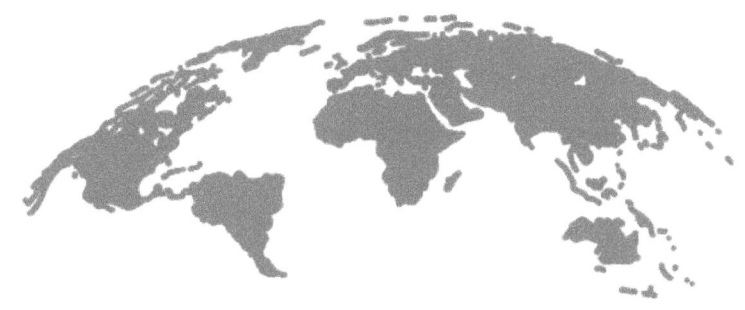

Evaluating possible dentists

Use the these pages to organize your research about one or more possible dentists (substituting your own priorities as needed).

EVALUATE PRACTICE

QUALITIES	DENTIST 1	DENTIST 2	DENTIST 3
NAME/ CONTACT DETAILS			
LOCATION/ DISTANCE			
FEES/ INSURANCE			
EXTRA GENTLE			
LIBERAL WITH PAINKILLERS			
CONSERVATIVE WITH INTERVENTIONS			
BIOLOGICAL, FUNCTIONAL, INTEGRATED			
SPECIAL EQUIPMENT			
SPECIAL MATERIALS			
SPECIAL SERVICES			
NOTES			

Draw on information from the dentist's website, discussions with friends, online reviews, speaking to the receptionist etc.

EVALUATE REPUTATION

QUALITIES	DENTIST 1	DENTIST 2	DENTIST 3
RECOMMENDED BY_____ BECAUSE_____			
IS THE DENTIST KNOWN TO BE OPEN-MINDED ABOUT PATIENT REQUESTS?			
DOES THE DENTIST HAVE A REPUTATION AS A GOOD LISTENER?			
HAS ANYBODY SAID THAT THE DENTIST DOESN'T EXPLAIN THEIR DECISIONS OR TAKES ACTIONS WITHOUT CONSENT FIRST			
IS THIS THE KIND OF DENTIST WHO WOULD BE WILLNG TO ADJUST THEIR OFFICE PRACTICES TO MEET NON-STANDARD NEEDS?			
NOTES			

PREPARE FOR THE CHAIR

In this section, the activities focus on preparing and practicing techniques you can use to relax and stay calm while work is being done in your mouth. Even if you don't do any of the preparation activities, the following activities may make all the difference to your dental experience.

Choose from a menu of simple, practical suggestions that have been proven to ease anxiety while patients stay still for dental procedures.

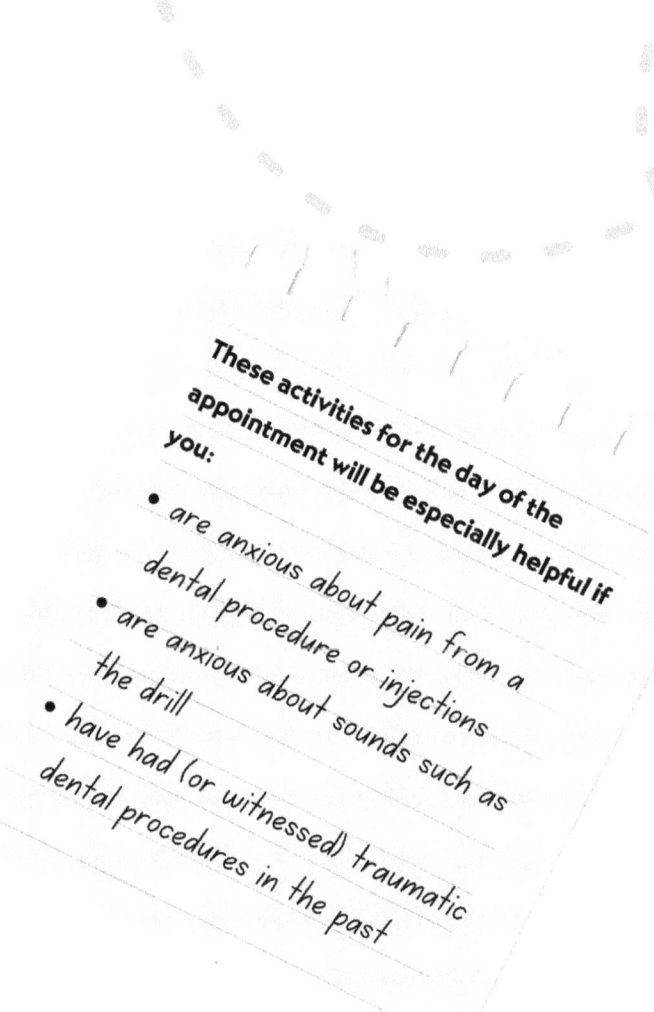

These activities for the day of the appointment will be especially helpful if you:

- are anxious about pain from a dental procedure or injections
- are anxious about sounds such as the drill
- have had (or witnessed) traumatic dental procedures in the past

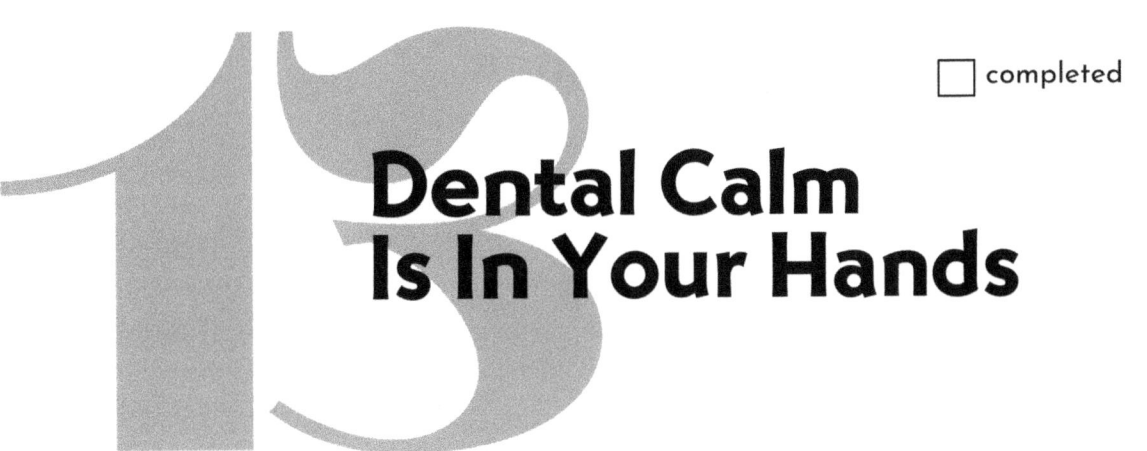

□ completed

Dental Calm Is In Your Hands

Many people find that a very effective strategy for staying calm in the dental chair is to focus on creating sensations in your hands. This is a way to stay still during a procedure without either spacing out or getting overwhelmed by what's being done inside your mouth.

Your mouth (and jaw) and your fingers (and hands) both contain some of the most concentrated networks of nerve endings in your body. The inside of your hands (palms and fingers) are almost as sensitive as the inside of your mouth.

That's why, when you focus your attention on sensations in your hands, the nerve receptors in your brain can get distracted from the sensations in your mouth.

The suggestions that follow might seem similar to forms of 'stimming' which is a coping strategy used by some people on the autism spectrum: repetitive motions or behaviors to help with sensory overload, alleviate anxiety or manage strong emotions.

In the following activities, the motions are very small and gentle so that your head and mouth won't move during a dental procedure. If you are someone who typically self-soothes with large or jerky stimming movements, it could take some practice to be able to get the benefits from these dental-friendly versions (or they may not be an option for you at all).

The following activities offer three ways to focus on your hands instead of your mouth and may be especially helpful if you:

- are very sensitive to pain, discomfort or sensory overload
- get emotionally triggered or energetically activated by someone working inside your mouth.

Hold onto something small

It can be really helpful to put something small in your pocket that you can pull out and hold in the dental chair such as a smooth crystal or other meaningful talisman.

I have an old seed and bead bracelet that I always wear to the dentist so I can rub the beads between my fingertips, letting its different textures help to keep me grounded. I discovered its calming effect when I was living in the Daintree Rainforest in Far North Queensland, Australia. I bought it for a few dollars at a craft market while waiting to have an emergency root canal with a dentist I'd never met before. Since then I've restrung it onto new elastic at least three times because I value its soothing qualities so much.

Brainstorm some ideas for a small object or piece of jewellery with comforting associations, that would be interesting to hold onto in the dental chair. Do you own something like this? Could you find, buy or borrow something to hold?

Hold onto another person

Human touch can be the most comforting support, so if you have a lot of anxiety, it might be helpful to ask a family member or friend to come along and hold your hand. I recommend letting the dental team know in advance if you are planning to hold hands with your support person during the procedure, so that it's not something that has to be explained and negotiated during your appointment.

How do you feel about asking someone to come along and hold your hand?

Who would be the best person to ask to come along and hold your hand?

Who might be available?

When will you ask them?

Would you like them to look at any sections of this book

before they accompany you to the dentist?

What's your plan to let your dental team know

that you are bringing someone to hold your hand?

If the dental assistant or nurse is friendly and feels safe, you can ask them to hold your hand during the procedure.

TIP

Stroke your fingers together

If another person's hand isn't available or isn't what you want, stroking your own hands together in very small movements that don't make your head shift around is almost as good.

This is a powerful self-soothing technique that you can do in the dental chair to help calm your mind, soothe strong emotions and stay still when you feel restless.

Try it now by placing both your hands over your belly
with the tips of your fingers resting
against the inside of the opposite hand.

Slowly and gently stroke the tips of your fingers
along the length of the fingers of your opposite hands.

Do this repeatedly,
curling your fingers each time
so that your wrists don't move.

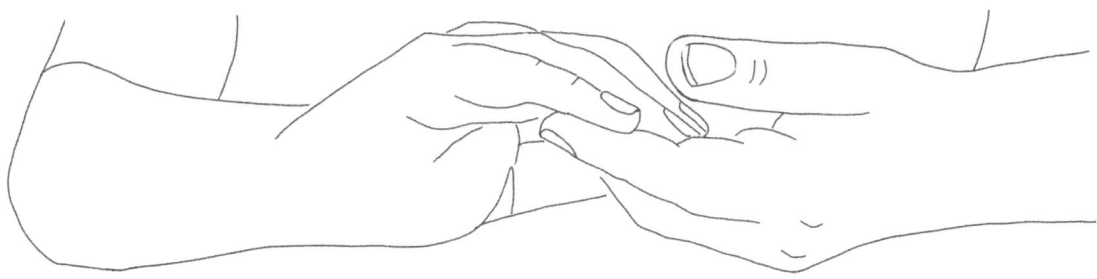

This kind of soothing touch releases relaxing hormones from the brain.

It is inspired by Havening Techniques, which use therapeutic touch to change the pathways in your brain that are linked with emotional distress. Havening Techniques were developed by a dentist, Dr Steven Rudin (with his twin brother Ronald) who used it to help his patients with dental phobias and traumas*.

It is simple and safe to do in the dental chair if you use very small, slow movements that won't interfere with your dental team's work. Havening Techniques may also be helpful to practice while you are doing some of the other activities in this book. Whenever you notice that you don't feel safe, try lightly stroking the tops of your arms, the outside of your face and the palms of your hands together to self soothe.

Try wriggling, flexing or rubbing your toes together in small movements that don't shift your head or mouth.

Try focusing on pelvic floor exercises without moving your body at all.

Can you think of any other ways to focus on your hands or another part of your body without moving your head or mouth?

*Youngson, Robin, *Time to Heal: Better me, Better world*, Rebel Heart (2020)

☐ completed

14 Focus On Breathing

A fundamental practice for calming anxiety in any context is to focus on your breath, especially breathing through your nose. In this activity you can practice breathing slowly through your nostrils while your mouth is wide open. This technique comes in handy during a procedure that you don't like, such as an injection or drilling.

Your breath is always accessible and with practice and intention it can remain under your control even when you can do almost nothing else in the dental chair but endure. However, if you are someone who finds that focusing on your breath actually increases you anxiety, then this activity is not for you!

Slow, steady nasal breathing activates the parasympathetic nervous system, which reduces anxiety. It can take some concentration to breathe through your nose while your mouth is open, so that's why you're going to practice it now.

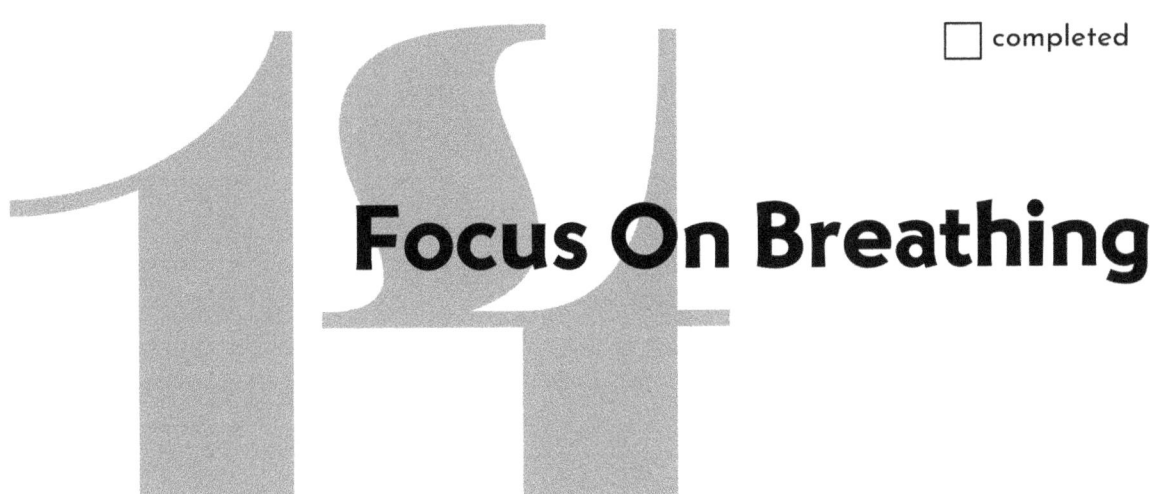

The following activities may be especially helpful if you:

- have difficulty breathing through your nose
- sometimes forget to breathe through your nose
- feel anxious about particular dental procedures
- have a lengthy, complicated dental surgery coming up.

PLEASE NOTE that breathing with your mouth (even if you are inhaling and exhaling through your nose) is not a healthy habit for your teeth and gums (because it dries out the oral microbiome) so only use this technique in the dental chair, or for dental prep.

Try syncing up your slow steady nose breathing with the slow gentle movement of your fingers stroking each other from Activity 13.

Breath work has been of such use to me, especially the mantra 'So Hum' which is just magic. On the in breath silently say 'So' and on the out breath, silently say 'Hum' and you remain calm through anything. Got me through my MRI and CT scans during investigations for oral cancer. I suffer from claustrophobia but by focusing on the So Hum mantra, I was chilled and calm.
—Morag Egan

Try syncing up your slow steady nose breathing with one of the visualizations in Activity 15.

TIP
It's easier to breathe through your nostrils if you blow your nose before practicing this activity, and before you get in the dental chair on the day.

Practice nose breathing
with your mouth open

Get ready to focus on your breathing by reclining back into some cushions to practice relaxing in a similar posture to being in the dental chair.

Once you are leaning back, open your mouth wide while you breathe through your nose. Concentrate on the feeling of air entering and leaving your nostrils.

Let the back of your tongue block your throat so air is directed only through your nose.

Making your out-breath last a little longer than your in-breath helps your body to relax even more.

Take a slow breath in, feel your belly rise,
and count 1, 2, 3, 4...

Make a slow breath out, and feel your belly fall,
counting 1, 2, 3, 4, 5...

Repeat with a slow in-breath as your belly rises
1, 2, 3, 4...

and a slow out-breath, as your belly falls,
1, 2, 3, 4, 5...

☐ completed

15 Prepare Your Mind

This activity is about giving your mind a job to do during your dental procedure so that you are less likely to think about worries or discomfort. Plan ahead with something pleasant to think about, especially if your thoughts tend to spiral into anxiety or negativity when not engaged elsewhere.

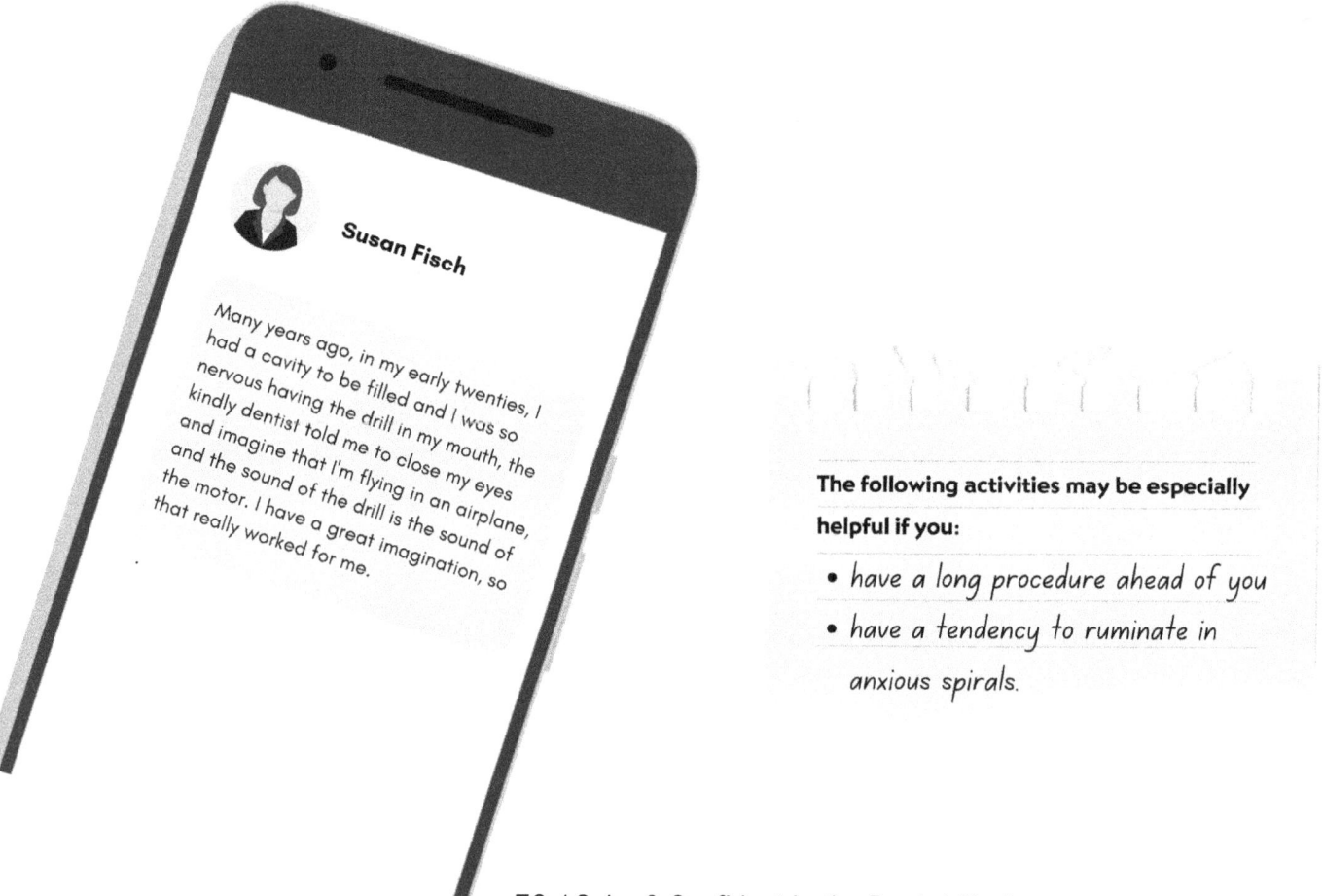

Susan Fisch

Many years ago, in my early twenties, I had a cavity to be filled and I was so nervous having the drill in my mouth, the kindly dentist told me to close my eyes and imagine that I'm flying in an airplane, and the sound of the drill is the sound of the motor. I have a great imagination, so that really worked for me.

The following activities may be especially helpful if you:

- have a long procedure ahead of you
- have a tendency to ruminate in anxious spirals.

If visualization works for you, it may be powerful to picture images that are metaphors or analogies for your body supporting the procedure you're going through. It doesn't need to be a complex image. Simple repetition can be very effective. The more vivid your visualization, the more your body can support the procedure.

Here are some ideas using nature imagery. Feel free to adapt and enhance them to be more resonant with what feels good and meaningful to you.

During an examination or x-ray:

Visualize midday sun beams shining down
through a broadleaf tree,
highlighting every detail of the veins of the leaves
and illuminating all the complexities of the forest ecosystem.
Feel the bright warmth of the sun on your skin with pleasure.

During a cleaning:

Visualize yourself scraping moss off of a stone wall,
imagine the movement of your hands holding a scraper,
feel the moss and lichen separating easily from the stones.

During injections:

Visualize cooling off in a refreshing sun shower,
imagine enjoying raindrops sparkling in the sunshine
and creating little rainbows
as they sprinkle lightly onto your skin.
Feel how your pores open up to drink in
the delightful moisture.
Smell the unique ozone scent of rain on a hot dry day.

During drilling:

Visualize digging into garden soil
in preparation for sowing seeds.
Feel how the soil gives way under your spade,
smell the life in the sweet rich earth under your feet,
see the healthy life living underground.

During a filling:

Visualize planting healthy seedlings in soft damp, fertile soil,
where the roots immediately take hold firmly.
Imagine patting the earth into place around each little plant,
sprinkling them with fresh water
and watching the seedlings stretch up towards the light.

During an extraction:

Visualize effortlessly pulling a ripe carrot out of soft soil,
feel the tug of the root giving way easily,
see the healthy space it leaves behind
filling with underground life.

During an implant, root canal or graft:

Visualize planting a strong sapling,
imagine its roots being welcomed
by all the creatures of the soil.

Take a moment now to think of a pleasant, life-affirming metaphor that is even more meaningful to you than any of my suggestions, one which also reflects what is planned for your next dental appointment.

Draw or describe this metaphor here and explore how you can engage with it using as many of your five senses as possible.

TIP

I don't recommend relying solely on visualisation to get you through a dental procedure safely and comfortably, especially if your body has a history of reacting badly to invasive treatments.

However, once you have made an informed decision and prepared as much as possible to minimize risks, you could try visualizing protective, resilient imagery such as sparkly armour, a spacious moat or a buoyant life jacket.

More ideas for positive thinking

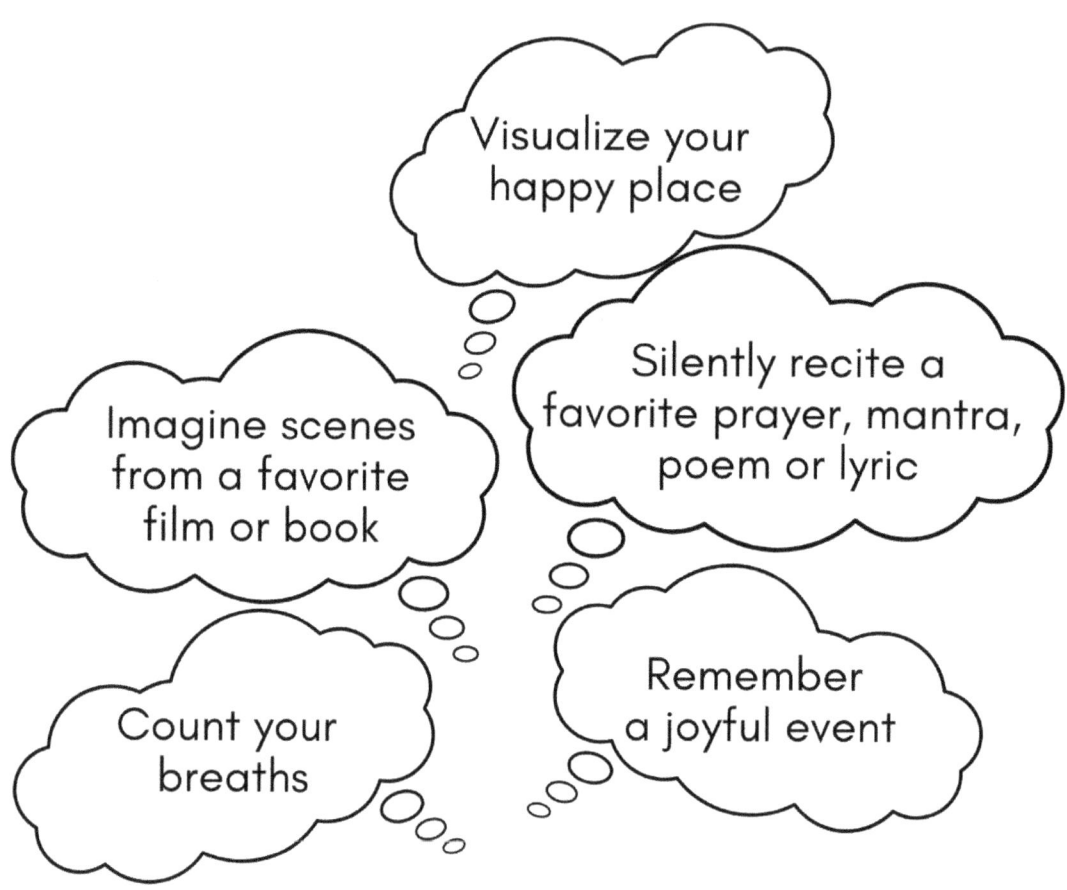

Make a plan for thinking positive and helpful thoughts during your next dental procedure.

☐ completed

16 Prepare Your Ears (And Eyes)

Dental tools can be very noisy and dentists need bright lights to see inside your mouth. Dentistry's distinctive sights, and sounds in particular, can activate uncomfortable feelings ranging from fear to being overwhelmed.

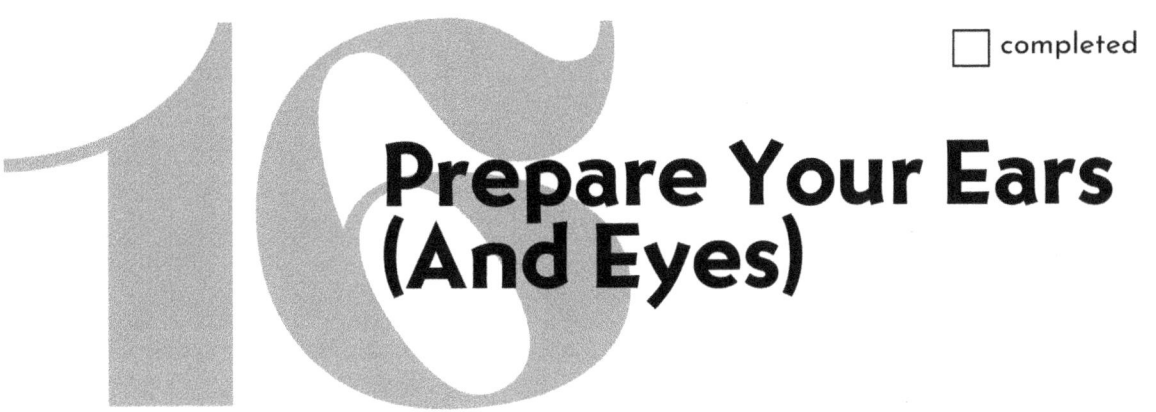

The following activities may be especially helpful if you:

- *get triggered or activated by the sound of the drill*
- *are highly sensitive or neurodivergent.*

Pick the activities that fit with your own needs or preferences.

To block bright lights

Consider wearing a sleep mask or sunglasses if the dental clinic's bright lights are uncomfortable or overstimulating for you. Add these to the list of *Things to Bring* in Activity 4.

If appropriate, tell your dentist that you are sensitive to the lights, so they can be extra careful to keep them from shining into your eyes as much as possible. Add this as a note to your list of *Intentions and Boundaries* in Activity 12, and practice talking to your dental team about it in Activity 19.

To drown out the drill

Do you want to create a music playlist to help distract you from the procedure while you listen on a smart phone (or other device) and headphones or earbuds? That way you'll be able to hear your music even if the dental tools are making a lot of noise.

If you are just going in for a check-up, playing your own music may not be necessary or convenient. Check-up tools aren't usually noisy and don't take much time. Check-ups can also be quite conversational (depending on how chatty your dentist is) meaning that it's often easier not to have anything playing in your ears.

For lengthy procedures, make sure you line up a long enough playlist to last for your whole session.

Avoid running out of music and wishing you could stop everything to fiddle with your phone midway through an appointment. Before you sit in the dental chair, make sure you have turned off notifications on your device and if necessary, block ads on your playlist.

I really like to drown out the sound of drilling or scraping with loud music that has strong familiar melodies and not many quiet interludes.

Check out some of the songs on my Drown out the Drill playlist. (Can you tell I was a teen in the 1980s?)

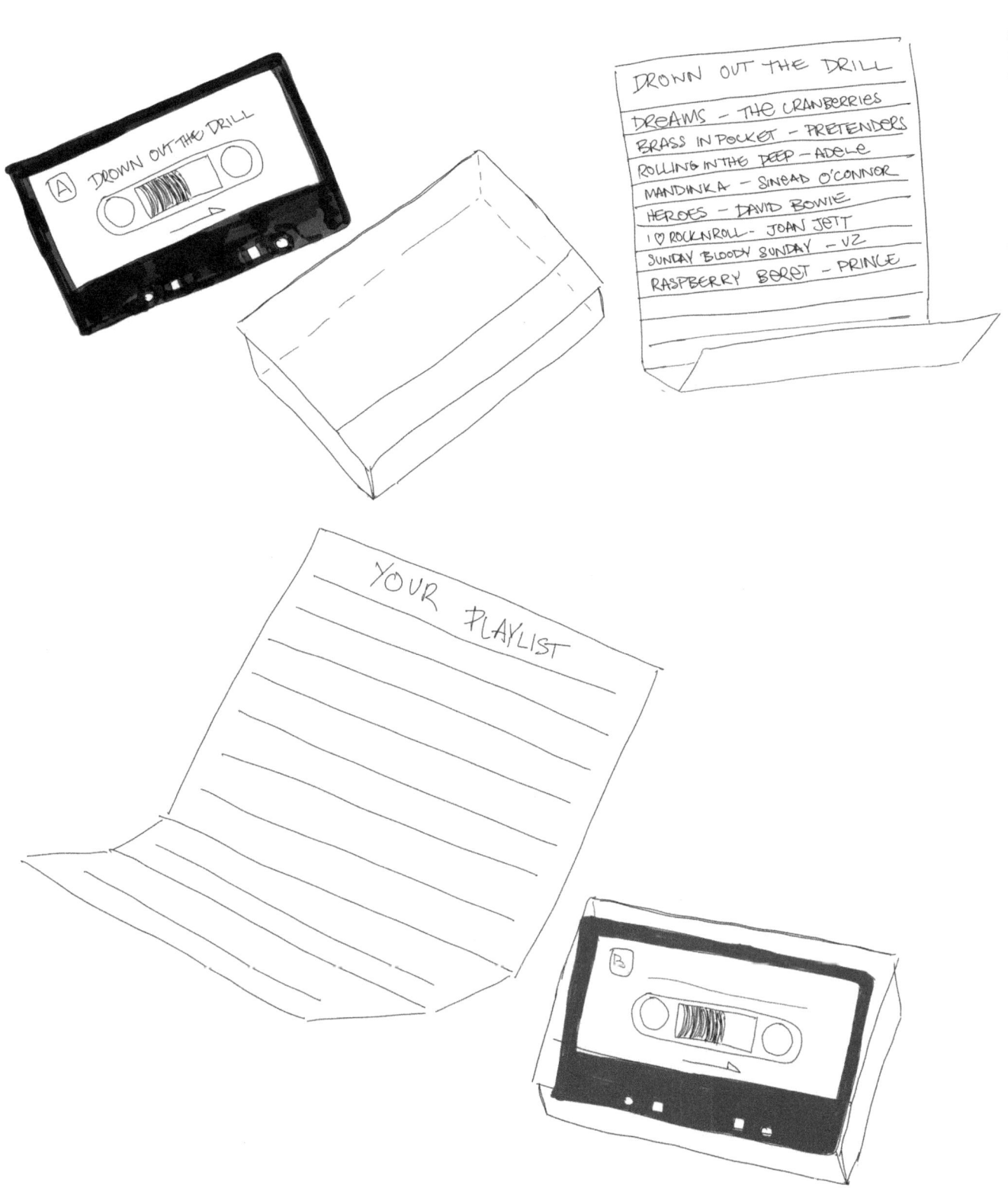

DROWN OUT THE DRILL

A DROWN OUT THE DRILL

DROWN OUT THE DRILL

DREAMS – THE CRANBERRIES
BRASS IN POCKET – PRETENDERS
ROLLING IN THE DEEP – ADELE
MANDINKA – SINEAD O'CONNOR
HEROES – DAVID BOWIE
I ♡ ROCK N ROLL – JOAN JETT
SUNDAY BLOODY SUNDAY – U2
RASPBERRY BERET – PRINCE

YOUR PLAYLIST

B

Write ideas for songs that you would like on your playlist here.

To minimize sounds

Bring along noise cancelling headphones or earbuds to use after you have finished your initial conversation with the dental team. Add these to the list of *Things to Bring* in Activity 4.

Explain to your dentist or hygienist that you'll be using noise-cancelling headphones, so that they know to get your attention with a hand signal or light touch if needed.

Would it be helpful to tell your dentist that you are sensitive to noise? Specify whether you are bothered by noise in general or just by particular sounds.

You might want to ask the dental team to:
- turn off any music that is playing in the background,
- keep the office door closed to block sounds from the rest of the building,
- avoid talking to you during a procedure unless absolutely necessary, or
- keep cross-talk among the dental team to a minimum.

Add your needs about noise to your list of *Intentions and Boundaries* in Activity 12, and practice talking to your dental team about it in Activity 19.

COMMUNICATE CONFIDENTLY

In this section, the activities will help you to prepare for clear, empowered and empathic communication with your team of dental professionals. The activities may help you to ask questions or explain your symptoms so that your dentist can understand exactly what you mean, and help you understand exactly what they say.

It can feel disempowering to be lying back in the dental chair, and submitting to invasive, uncomfortable or humiliating treatment. A sense of powerlessness can be overwhelming, especially if you feel:

- unacknowledged
- that the dental team members are speaking to each other as though you aren't there
- you can't make yourself understood (especially while work is underway in your mouth).

Dental professionals have a responsibility to do whatever is possible to support good communication with their patients.

Some of them are better at it than others, and there's a limit to how much influence you can have over your dental team's communication skills and style.

However, you can do a lot to set the tone for good communication when you explain your intentions and boundaries at the start of your appointment.

What you bring to the conversation matters a great deal. Therefore, try to:

- get clear about what you want to say before the appointment (Activities 10, 11, 17 and 22)

- practice using empowered body language during the appointment (Activities 19 and 20)

- make an effort to be empathetic and understand the dental team's perspective (Activity 18).

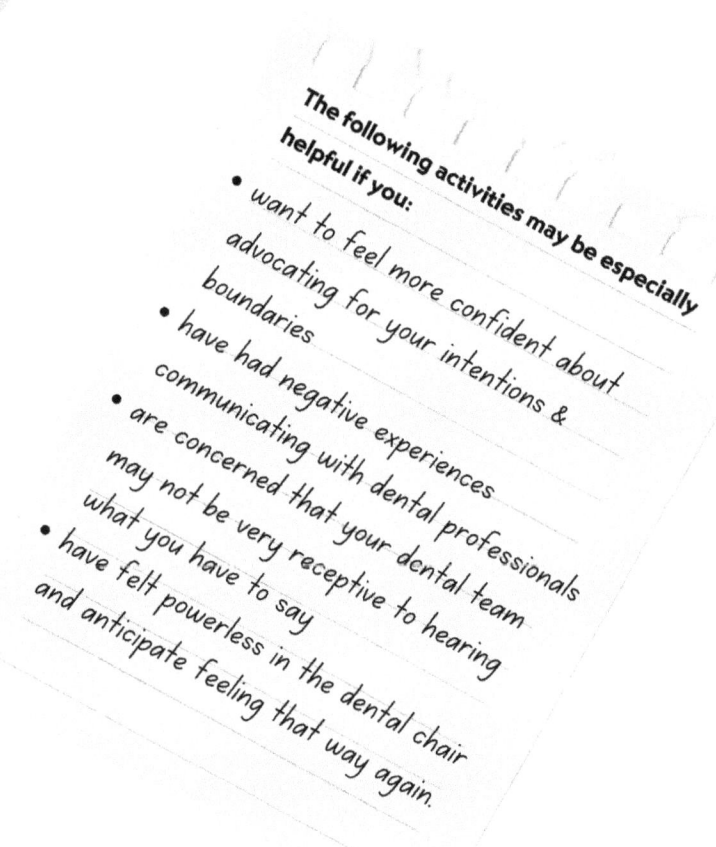

The following activities may be especially helpful if you:

- want to feel more confident about advocating for your intentions & boundaries

- have had negative experiences communicating with dental professionals

- are concerned that your dental team may not be very receptive to hearing what you have to say

- have felt powerless in the dental chair and anticipate feeling that way again.

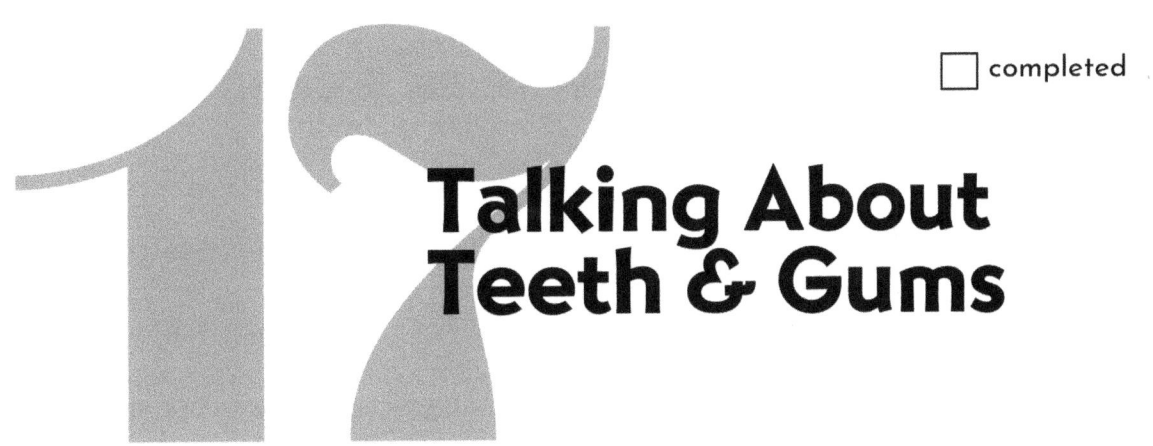

☐ completed

Talking About Teeth & Gums

This activity is intended to help you explain your symptoms or ask questions with more clarity, and to better understand what your dental team is talking about.

The dental profession uses varying words (and numbers) to describe the same things depending on where they practice (or where your dentist was trained). It can be confusing!

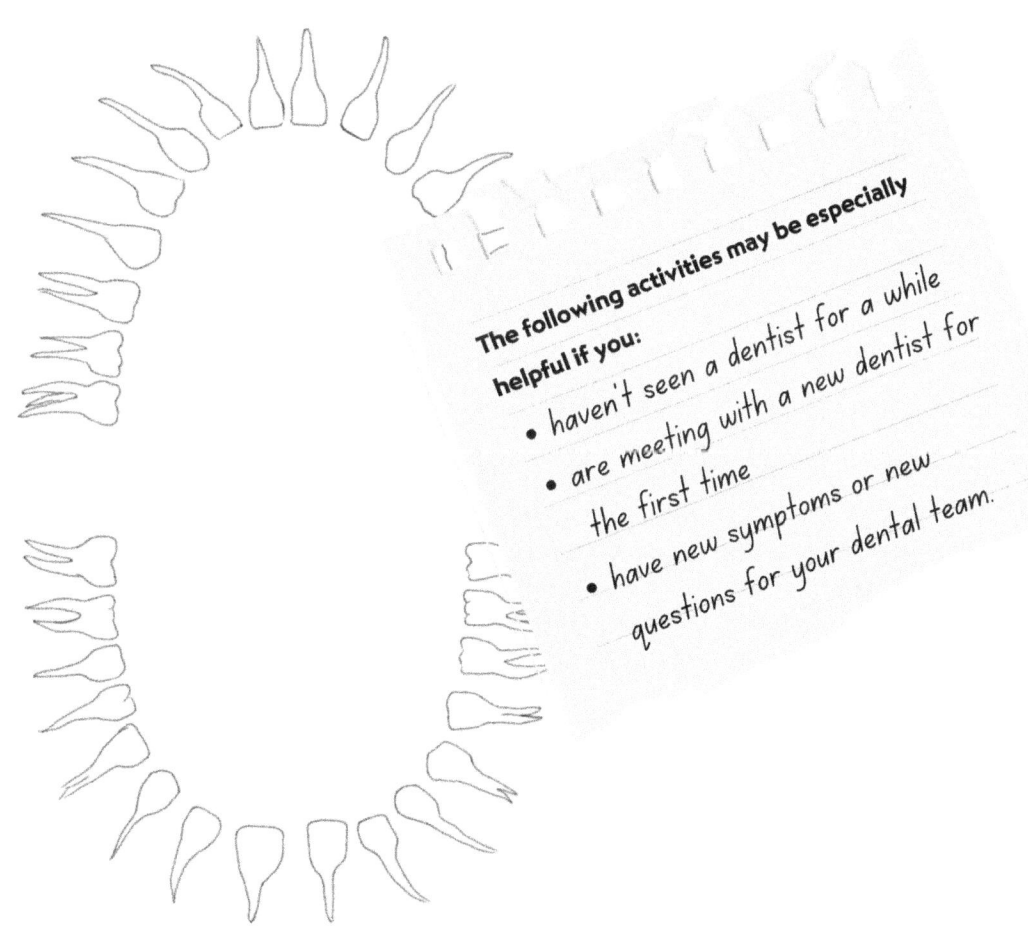

The following activities may be especially helpful if you:

- haven't seen a dentist for a while
- are meeting with a new dentist for the first time
- have new symptoms or new questions for your dental team.

Explaining your observations & concerns

Prepare for your next dental appointment by making note of any symptoms you've noticed with your teeth or gums such as:

- sensitivity or pain

- receding, bleeding or swollen gums

- changes to the colors of your teeth, gums, tongue, palate or inside of cheeks

- teeth that are moving or loose, or your bite changing

- tight or sore jaw

- clenching or grinding teeth

- any lesions, lumps or swollen lymph nodes on your mouth, face or neck

- bad breath or a bad taste in your mouth.

Make a note of any general health concerns, diagnoses, or significant life events that have caused stress since your last dental appointment

When did you last see a dental professional and what did they recommend?

SYMPTOM NOTES

SYMPTOM	LOCATION	FIRST NOTICED & HOW OFTEN	INTENSITY	NOTES & CONCERNS

Navigating names and numbers

It's helpful to know the names and numbers of your teeth that need attention, especially if there is more than one area of your mouth with problems. However, when you switch to a new dentist, are referred to a specialist or speak with an oral health coach like me, you might find that we each use different names and numbers to refer to the same teeth.

UPPER TEETH

TOOTH TYPE	POSITION	UNIVERSAL	FDI	PALMER
WISDOM, THIRD MOLAR	UPPER RIGHT BACK	1	18	8 ⌐
SECOND MOLAR	UPPER RIGHT BACK	2	17	7 ⌐
FIRST MOLAR	UPPER RIGHT SIDE	3	16	6 ⌐
SECOND PREMOLAR, SECOND BICUSPID	UPPER RIGHT SIDE	4	15	5 ⌐
FIRST PREMOLAR, FIRST BICUSPID	UPPER RIGHT SIDE	5	14	4 ⌐
CANINE, CUSPID, EYE TOOTH	UPPER RIGHT FRONT	6	13	3 ⌐
LATERAL INCISOR	UPPER RIGHT FRONT	7	12	2 ⌐
CENTRAL INCISOR	UPPER RIGHT FRONT	8	11	1 ⌐
CENTRAL INCISOR	UPPER LEFT FRONT	9	21	⌐ 1
LATERAL INCISOR	UPPER LEFT FRONT	10	22	⌐ 2
CANINE, CUSPID, EYE TOOTH	UPPER LEFT FRONT	11	23	⌐ 3
FIRST PREMOLAR, FIRST BICUSPID	UPPER LEFT SIDE	12	24	⌐ 4
SECOND PREMOLAR, SECOND BICUSPID	UPPER LEFT SIDE	13	25	⌐ 5
FIRST MOLAR	UPPER LEFT SIDE	14	26	⌐ 6
SECOND MOLAR	UPPER LEFT BACK	15	27	⌐ 7
WISDOM, THIRD MOLAR	UPPER LEFT BACK	16	28	⌐ 8

Most dentists use one of three major numbering systems. The **Universal** numbering system is most common in the USA, and it's the one that I use in my books, on my website and with my clients. The World Health Organisation's **FDI** (ISO 3950) system is used internationally. The **Palmer** notation system is an older system still used commonly in the UK.

LOWER TEETH

TOOTH TYPE	POSITION	UNIVERSAL	FDI	PALMER
WISDOM, THIRD MOLAR	LOWER LEFT BACK	17	38	8⌐
SECOND MOLAR	LOWER LEFT BACK	18	37	7⌐
FIRST MOLAR	LOWER LEFT SIDE	19	36	6⌐
SECOND PREMOLAR, SECOND BICUSPID	LOWER LEFT SIDE	20	35	5⌐
FIRST PREMOLAR, FIRST BICUSPID	LOWER LEFT SIDE	21	34	4⌐
CANINE, CUSPID, EYE TOOTH	LOWER LEFT FRONT	22	33	3⌐
LATERAL INCISOR	LOWER LEFT FRONT	23	32	2⌐
CENTRAL INCISOR	LOWER LEFT FRONT	24	31	1⌐
CENTRAL INCISOR	LOWER RIGHT FRONT	25	41	⌐1
LATERAL INCISOR	LOWER RIGHT FRONT	26	42	⌐2
CANINE, CUSPID, EYE TOOTH	LOWER RIGHT FRONT	27	43	⌐3
FIRST PREMOLAR, FIRST BICUSPID	LOWER RIGHT SIDE	28	44	⌐4
SECOND PREMOLAR, SECOND BICUSPID	LOWER RIGHT SIDE	29	45	⌐5
FIRST MOLAR	LOWER RIGHT SIDE	30	46	⌐6
SECOND MOLAR	LOWER RIGHT BACK	31	47	⌐7
WISDOM, THIRD MOLAR	LOWER RIGHT BACK	32	48	⌐8

Mark up the preceding tables to remind yourself which numbering system your dental team uses, and which of your teeth require attention at the moment.

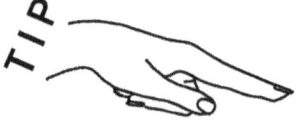

When talking about locations inside your mouth, right and left always refer to *your* right and left, not the dentist's! Note that all the numbering systems include wisdom teeth.

Another way of keeping track of your teeth is with a map or diagram of the mouth. This format may be particularly useful if you retain information better in a visual format.

You can use this mouth map (with Universal numbers) to draw or write notes about your symptoms and other observations.

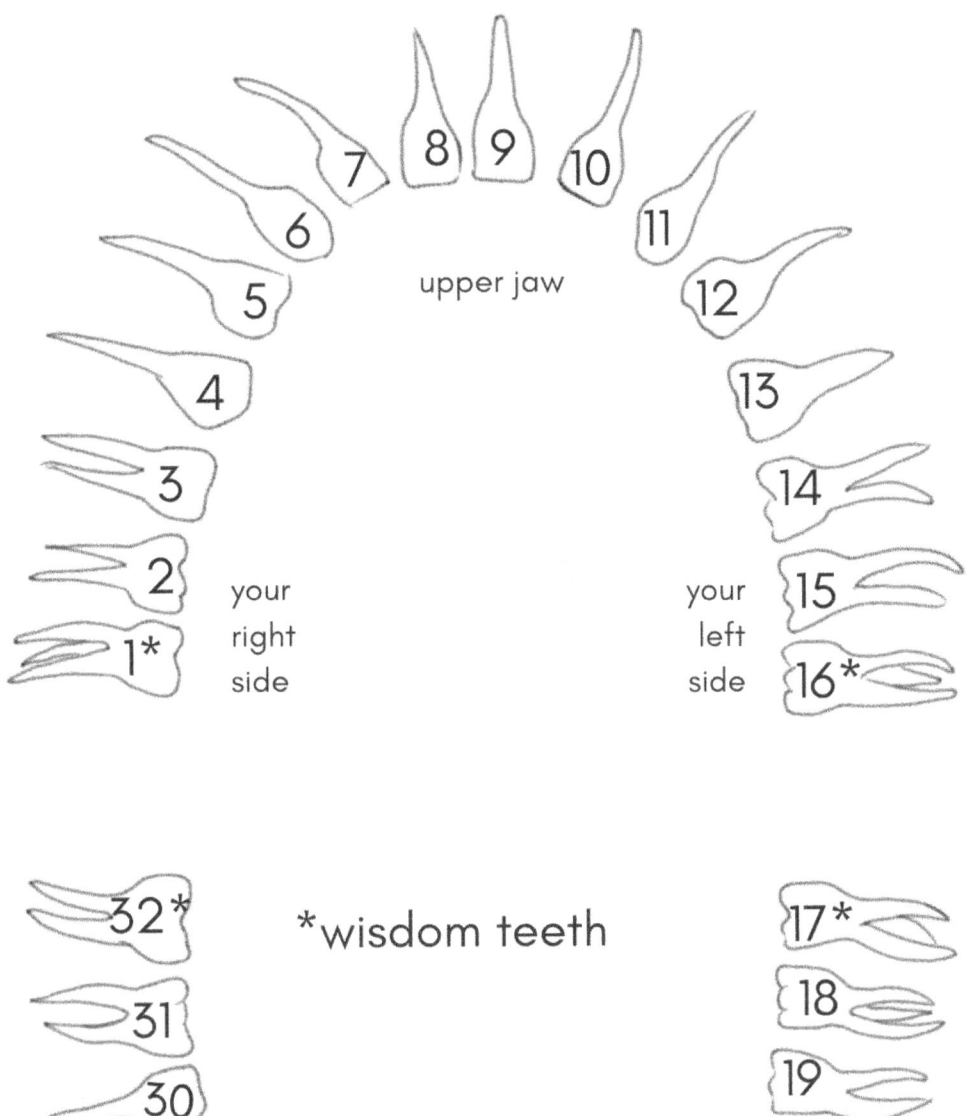

upper jaw

7 8 9 10

6 11

5 12

4 13

3 14

2 15

your right side   your left side

1*   16*

32*   *wisdom teeth   17*

31   18

30   19

29   20

28   21

27   22

26   lower jaw   23

25 24

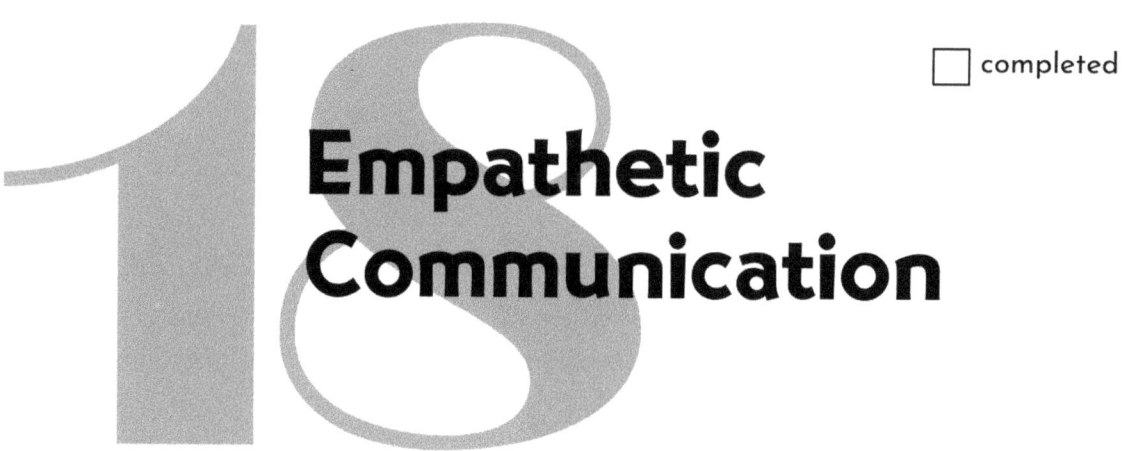

Empathetic Communication

In this visualization activity, the focus is on wishing your dental team well and visualizing (perhaps manifesting) the best possible interactions with them.

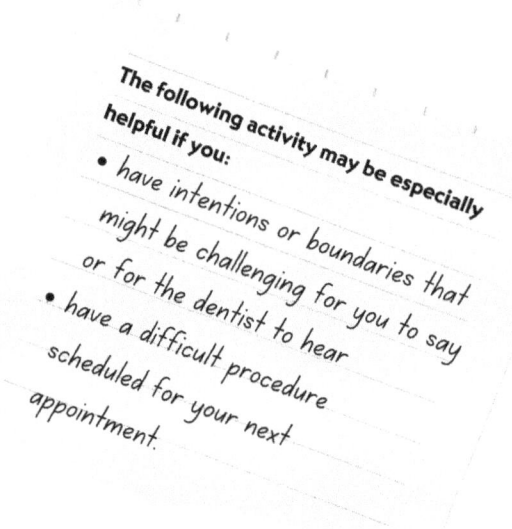

The following activity may be especially helpful if you:

- have intentions or boundaries that might be challenging for you to say or for the dentist to hear
- have a difficult procedure scheduled for your next appointment.

Every day your dentist spends hours getting up close to people who may not want to see them, and who may be resistant (and perhaps highly emotional) about being there. One of the ways dentists cope with these pressures is by controlling the flow of each appointment.

When you do something unexpected like standing up (Activity 19) to talk through your intentions and boundaries (Activity 11), that could feel disconcerting for your dental team. You can help to make it easier for them to meet your needs if you imagine yourself in their shoes.

Dentists are human too, with just as many potential communication strengths and weaknesses as anyone else.

Your dentist was trained to feel confident in making definitive diagnoses and delivering technical solutions to all or most of your dental issues.

However, they may or may not have had much training in empathetic listening or trauma-informed communication. They are also often under pressure to work within tight timeframes that don't allow for lengthy conversations.

Most dentists want to be kind and compassionate.

Most dentists (in my recent experience) understand the importance of listening to patients respectfully. Most will do their best to accommodate your intentions and boundaries, even if it requires an unfamiliar approach. You won't know if you don't ask.

Dentists are working in one of the most feared and disliked professions. They are at more risk from exposure to infectious disease, radiation and heavy metals than many other health professionals. Dentists have one of the highest rates of work-related mental illness and suicide. Dental hygienists and dental assistants deal with many of the same challenges but at a much lower paygrade and with less control over their work.

Sometimes you might find yourself dealing with a dental professional who comes across as dismissive, disrespectful or arrogant. If your dentist consistently behaves in those ways, then you can and should take your business elsewhere. But if it's the first time they've acted this way they might just be having a bad day.

For the following visualization, download the audio recording in the bonus content (link on page 3) or read through the words, and then close your eyes and either picture each scene in your imagination or tell yourself each scene as a little story.

COMMUNICATION

First think about your dental team.
Say their names if you know them,
picture their faces if you remember what they look like,
or imagine kind, friendly humans for the purpose of this exercise.

Picture your dental team at home
on the night before your appointment
enjoying a peaceful evening,
with warm connections and relaxing activities.

Imagine your dentist asleep in bed,
deep in a night of restorative rest,
dreaming pleasant dreams of competence and success.

Imagine their unhurried, nourishing morning routine
and an uncomplicated trip to work on the day they see you.

Imagine that any earlier patients are easy and enjoyable
for the whole dental team.

Picture your team laughing companionably
so they are in a really good mood
and working together like a well-oiled machine.

Imagine how your dentist feels to be well rested,
well fed, happy, healthy,
competent, steady-handed, compassionate,
patient and open-minded
by the time your appointment rolls around.

Picture yourself opening the door to enter the dental practice
and seeing their smiling faces.

Imagine yourself greeting your dental team confidently
and then telling them everything they need to know
from your list of intentions and boundaries.

Make some notes about what you observed and felt during this visualization.

Try rewriting your intentions and boundaries from Activity 12 into a script using empathetic language.

Get a crush on your dentist

Some of the people I know who are the most enthusiastic about going for a dental appointment have (or have had) a little crush on their dentist.

Try paying attention to your dentist's attractive qualities and allowing yourself to feel some warm affection towards them. Of course, this should never be an excuse to say or do anything inappropriate to your professional relationship. But indulging in a mild and private crush might help overcome some of your resistance and dislike of sitting in the dental chair.

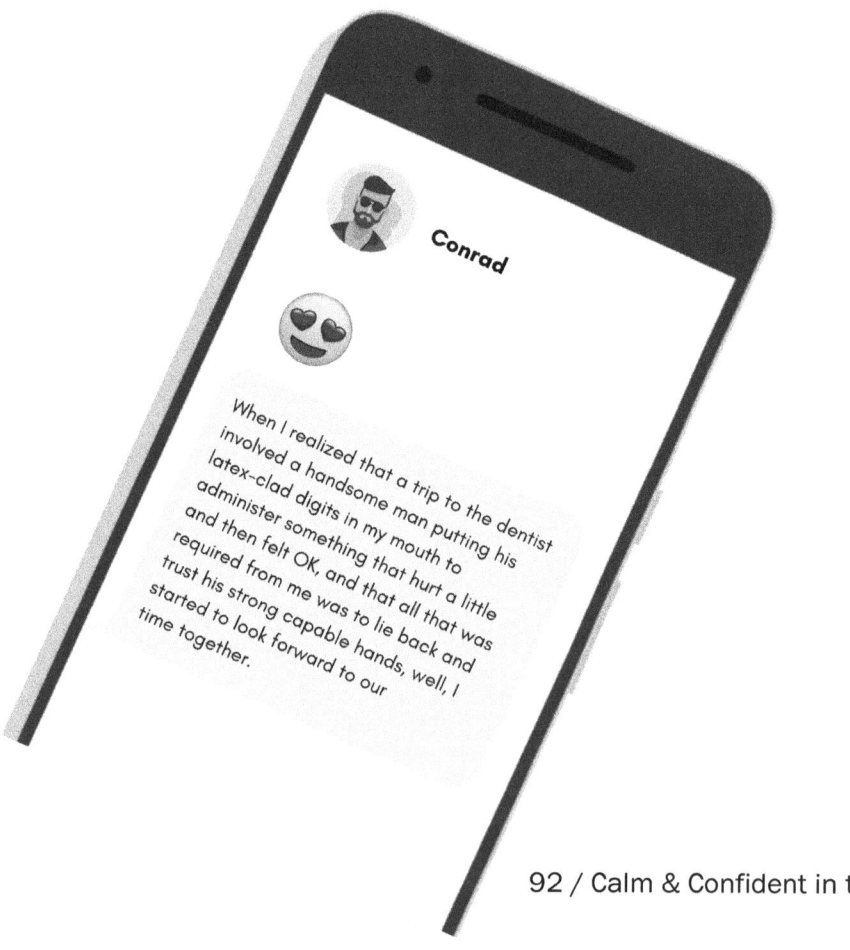

Conrad

😍

When I realized that a trip to the dentist involved a handsome man putting his latex-clad digits in my mouth to administer something that hurt a little and then felt OK, and that all that was required from me was to lie back and trust his strong capable hands, well, I started to look forward to our time together.

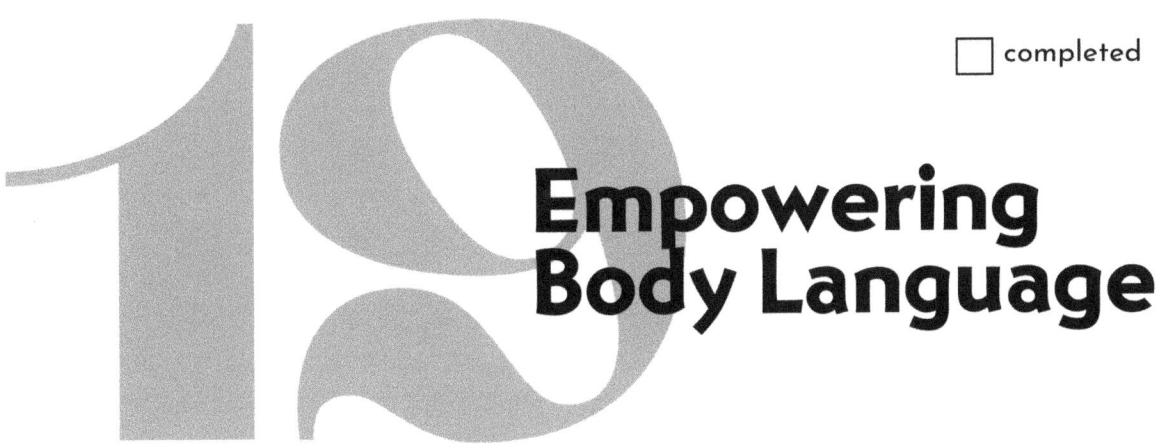

Empowering Body Language

☐ completed

This activity addresses a fundamental power imbalance found in most dentist-patient relationships.

One of the reasons that going to the dentist can feel so disempowering for some of us, may be connected to the ancient mammal-ancestor part of our brain. Lying belly up is a trusting and submissive posture for most animals. Think about the dogs and cats that you know. They only lie on their backs when they feel very safe.

When you lie on your back *despite feeling anxious*, it can create such an unconscious conflict that the discerning, independent-thinking part of your mind can shut down.

For some people, the sight and feeling of a dentist or hygienist leaning over you, probing inside your mouth makes that subconscious part of your brain feel threatened. It may be an irrational response, but it can be difficult to override the flood of hormones that activates a fight, flight, freeze (shut down) or fawn (self abandonment) response.

If you feel one or more of those responses while lying back in the dental chair, you could find yourself agreeing to procedures or tolerating discomfort that you would never go along with if you were standing upright.

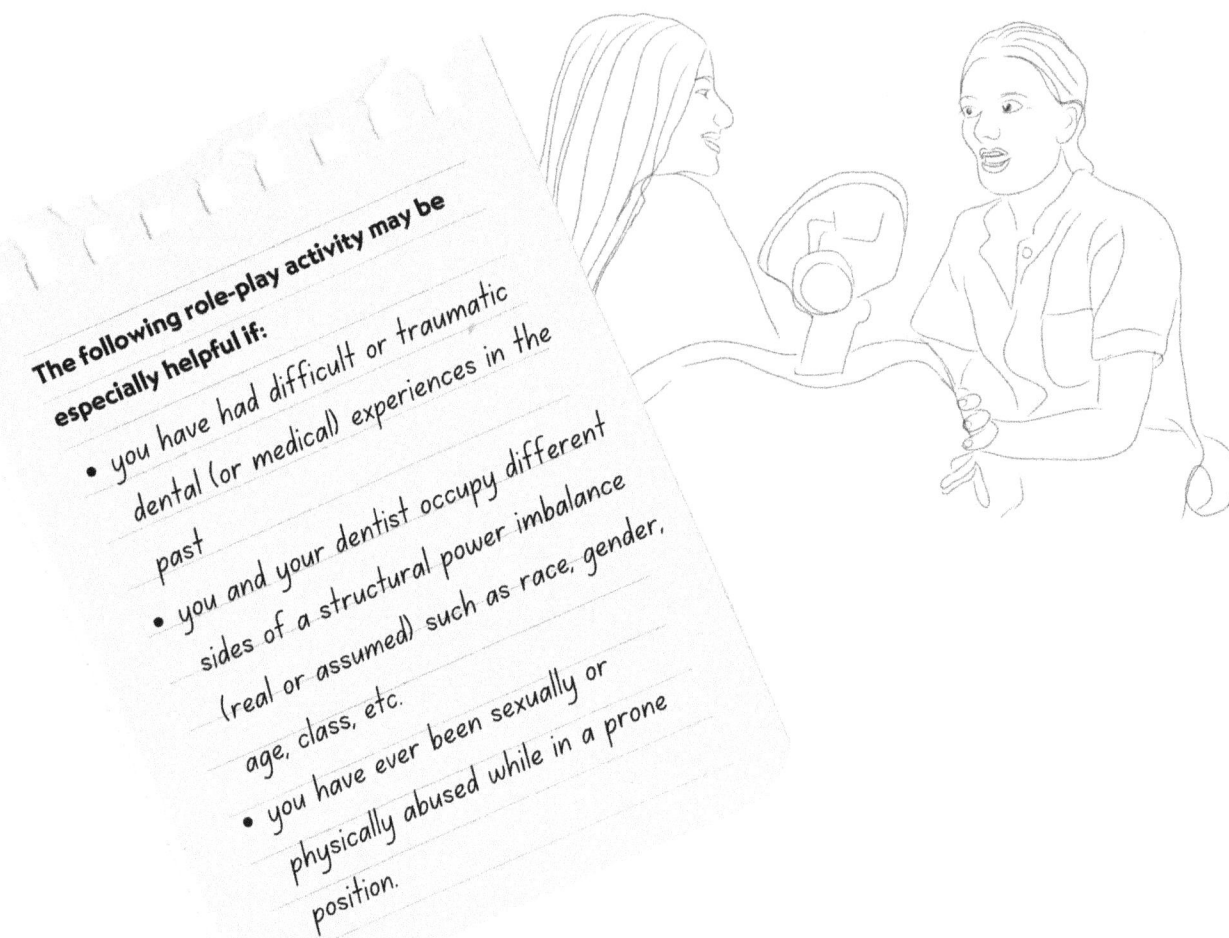

The following role-play activity may be especially helpful if:

- you have had difficult or traumatic dental (or medical) experiences in the past
- you and your dentist occupy different sides of a structural power imbalance (real or assumed) such as race, gender, age, class, etc.
- you have ever been sexually or physically abused while in a prone position.

Consider whether it would be helpful for you to sit upright or even stand up, for as much of the appointment as possible.

You only really need to be reclined while the dentist or hygienist is looking, or working, inside your mouth.

I like to perch on the side of the dental chair while talking rather than leaning back immediately.

You can stand up to greet the dental team at the beginning of the appointment. If appropriate, try setting the tone for empowering communication by shaking your dentist's hand and looking them in the eye. That's the body language used by equals in many cultures, including those cultures that dominate in the dental profession.

If possible, try standing or sitting upright while you say what you need to say to the team at the start of your appointment.

Role-play with a friend or family member to practice greeting and explaining your intentions and boundaries (from Activity 11) while sitting upright or standing. Children can often be enthusiastic role-play partners.

Use your script from Activity 18 to rehearse. Practice acting in both roles, as patient and as dentist. Having a turn as the dentist can help you better understand how the dental team may hear what you have to say.

If you don't have a role-play partner, you can practice on your own. Stand in front of a mirror, or sit upright in the car, to practice saying your piece in the same position you'll use to speak eye to eye in the dental office.

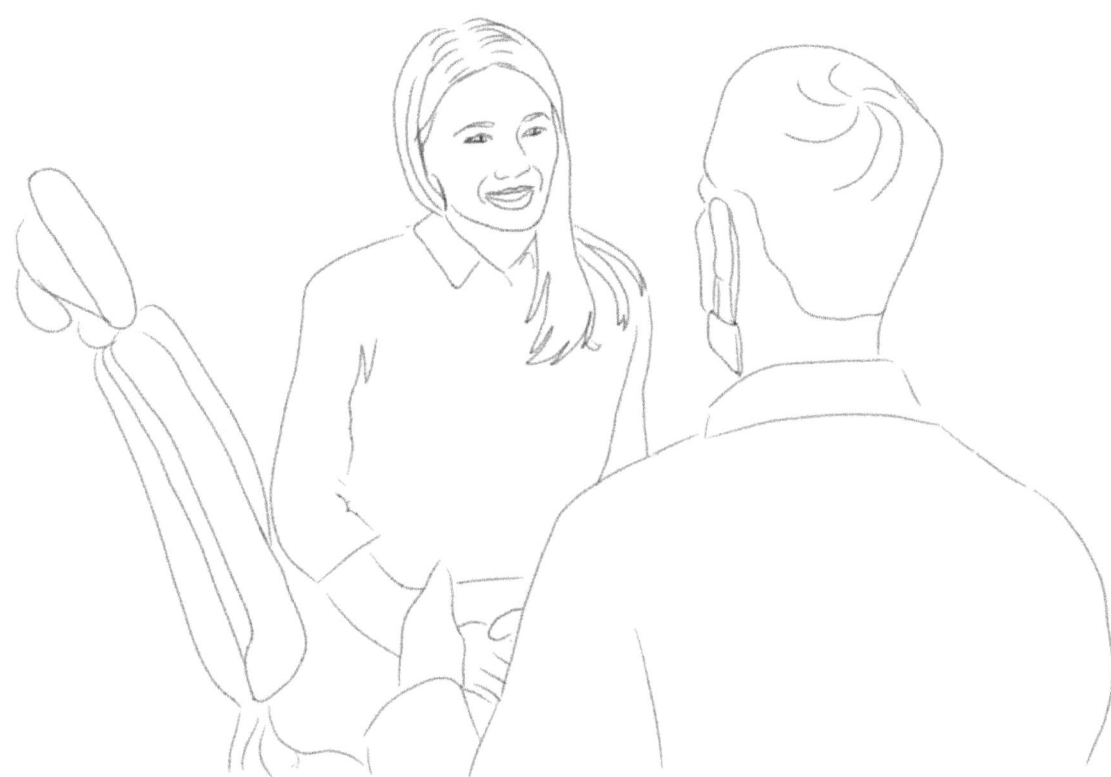

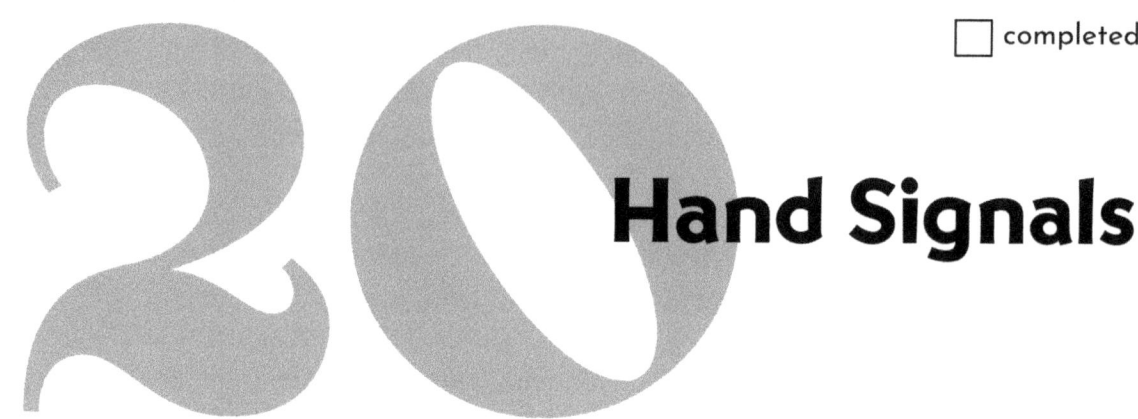

Hand Signals

No matter how busy the dental team seems to be doing things to the inside of your mouth, you're allowed to take a little breather during a procedure. Just lift your hand to signal the dentist to stop. If you have fixed equipment (like a dental dam) in your mouth, it may not be easy to talk but otherwise it's usually possible to ask a question or even get out of the chair to use the bathroom.

A good dentist will tell you to do this. Believe them. Really trusting that I could actually interrupt the dental team at work without negative consequences was key for me in getting over my dental anxiety.

This visualization activity may be especially helpful if you:

- feel trapped when you lie back in the dental chair
- are worried about pain, discomfort or sensory overload in the chair
- have a weak bladder and may need to get up during a procedure.

For the following visualization, download the audio recording in the bonus content (link on page 3) or read through the words, and then close your eyes and either picture the scene in your imagination or tell it to yourself as a little story.

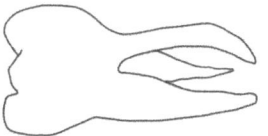

Imagine lying back in the dental chair,
feeling completely confident
that your needs and wishes have been heard respectfully
and will be accommodated to the best of the dentist's ability.

Imagine yourself reminding the dentist or hygienist
that you might lift your hand up to ask them to pause
while they are working inside your mouth.

Now imagine that during the procedure you do lift your hand.

Visualise the dentist willingly
bringing the chair upright to meet your needs,
then imagine lying back down comfortably again
so they can complete their work.

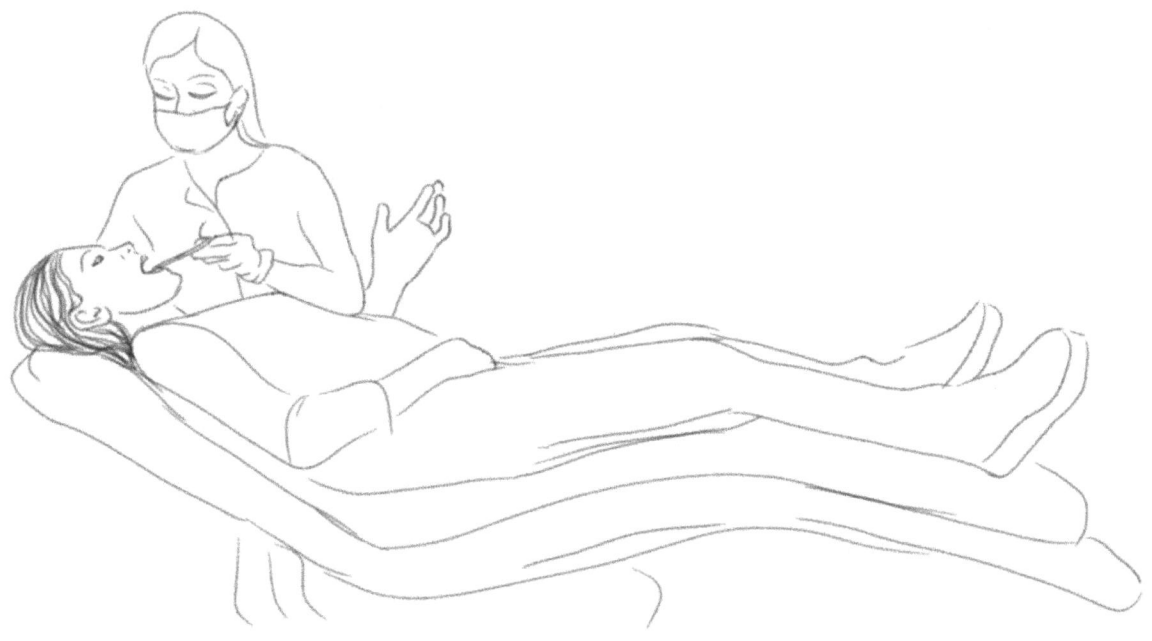

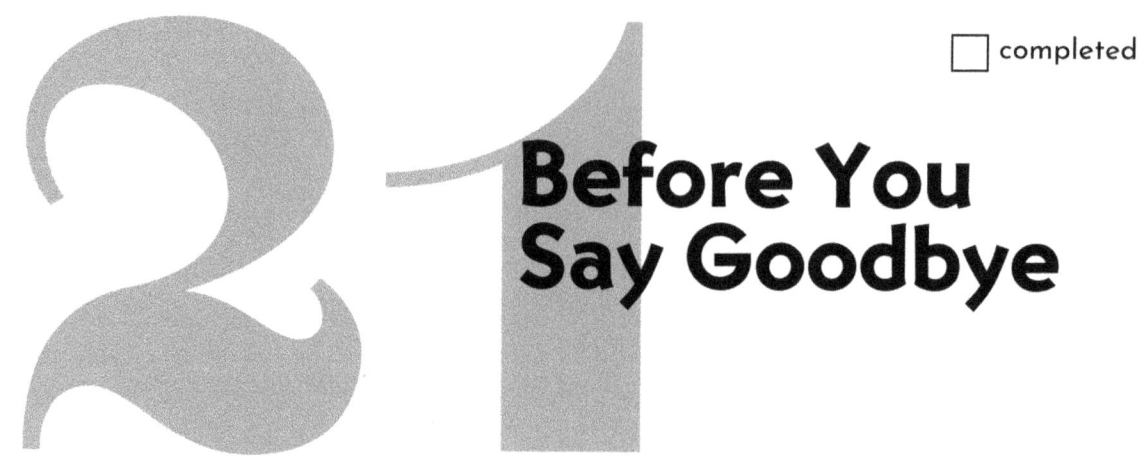

☐ completed

Before You Say Goodbye

Some of the most important communication from your dentist will happen after they've finished working inside your mouth, and before you leave.

At the end of your appointment, there can often be a lot of information for you to take in and you may be expected to make major decisions.

And yet that's a time when you could find it most difficult to listen, think and respond authentically. So, unless you are in a life-or-death dental emergency, you can postpone any decisions until you've had a chance to rest and recover.

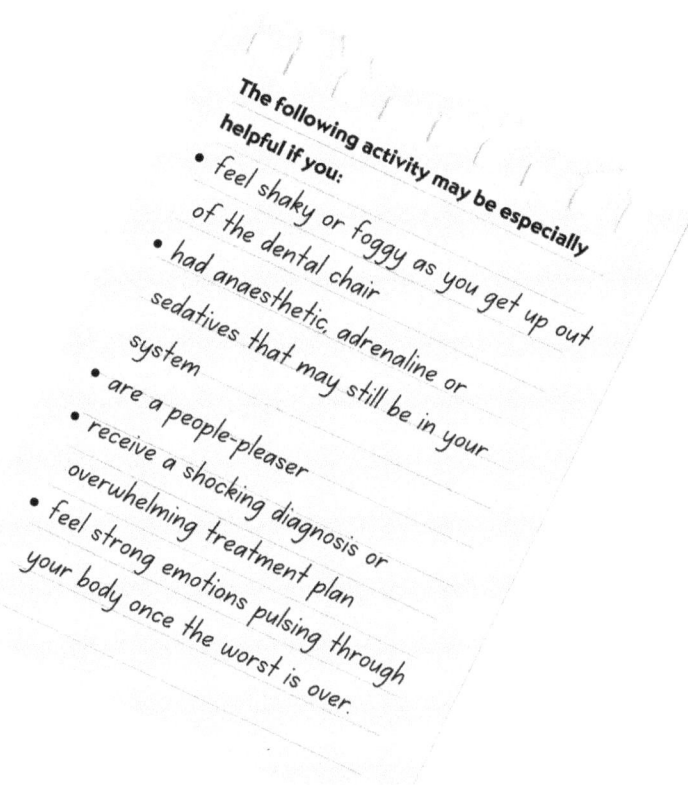

The following activity may be especially helpful if you:

- feel shaky or foggy as you get up out of the dental chair
- had anaesthetic, adrenaline or sedatives that may still be in your system
- are a people-pleaser
- receive a shocking diagnosis or overwhelming treatment plan
- feel strong emotions pulsing through your body once the worst is over.

Your dentist has two main tasks to complete after they finish your procedure and before they see the next patient or take a break. One is to talk to you and the other is to make their notes.

They'll often wait to make notes until you've left the room, but it's also common for dentists to make notes straight away, giving you a few moments to gather your wits before they report on the current state of your teeth and gums, or summarise the treatment they provided.

You can ask for a couple of extra minutes for a bathroom break, a stretch, some deep breaths, a drink of water or whatever you need to be more present for the conversation.

For the following visualization, download the audio recording in the bonus content (link on page 3) or read through the words, and then close your eyes and either picture the scene in your imagination or tell it to yourself as a little story.

Visualize yourself at the end of your appointment,
sitting back up in the chair.

Imagine asking for a little time to recover
before discussing the outcome with the dentist.

See yourself in the dental office taking a deep breath
and looking around.

Find something to focus your eyes on
that makes you feel safe:
maybe a picture on the wall or your coat hanging on a hook.
Imagine wriggling your fingers and toes, stretching your arms.

Now you are ready to listen to the dentist
with laser sharp attention,
asking the questions you need to fully understand
everything they are saying.

Imagine requesting
that they summarise their recommendations
or treatment plan in writing or as an email so you can consider
the information at your leisure, with a clear head.

Imagine yourself asking for copies
of any x-rays, CT scans or intraoral photographs.
See the dentist easily and happily agreeing to your requests.

Visualize yourself standing upright,
saying thank you and goodbye.

See yourself walking out of the dental office feeling good,
with the door closing behind you.
That's done now.

Imagine meeting with a friend afterwards
and telling them how good the dental appointment was,
how you spoke up for yourself
and how the dentist responded positively.

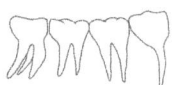

DIVE DEEPER

The preceding sections focused on giving you a tool kit to help prepare for your next dental appointment. In this chapter, you can explore the nuances and challenges of your dental ambivalence in more depth. If you have time, and inclination, you can do some of these exercises before your next appointment, but they are just as valuable to work through after the appointment.

There will always be more dental visits, and your goal of becoming calm and confident in the dental chair may take more than one session. Many of the activities in this section can be reviewed and practiced before every dental appointment.

These activities may be especially useful if you:

- received a complex treatment plan at your last dental appointment
- are considering a serious intervention such as a root canal, extraction, implant, graft, veneers or orthodontic treatment etc.
- have a long history of traumatic dental treatments
- tend to postpone dental appointments until you are in a crisis.

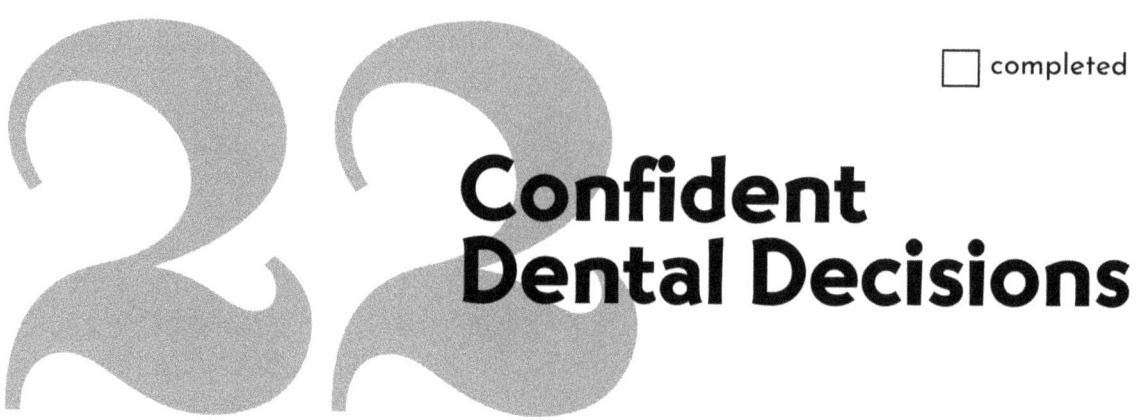

☐ completed

Confident Dental Decisions

Deciding whether, when and how to proceed with a dentist's advice can feel difficult, even more so if you are responsible for consenting on behalf of someone else (such as a child). In this activity, you'll focus on connecting with the wise inner part of you who already knows how to decide on your next step with a dental treatment plan.

These activities may be especially useful if you:
- have been advised to have a dental procedure that you aren't sure about, are scared of or can't afford
- have been postponing seeing the dentist because you don't want to hear what you think they will recommend
- received a contradictory second opinion from another dental or health professional
- thought you'd made up your mind about a treatment but new information or symptoms have you second-guessing yourself.

You can do the different parts of this activity all on the same day or in different sessions. You can bring it to a therapeutic conversation with someone you trust; or do it alone in a safe place. I recommend that you do the reorienting practice (Activity 2) to close each session whenever you stop, whether this exercise is completed or not.

Step 1. Information gathering

Brainstorm everything you know about the arguments in favor of the dentist's recommended treatment plan, why they think it's necessary and what the benefits would be of following this recommendation.

List any concerns, risks, fears and arguments against following that recommendation.

Now describe alternative(s), such as doing nothing or choosing a different procedure, or only doing one part of the treatment plan.

Do you have any questions that need to be answered before you can make an informed decision about your options? Use the table on this page to organise your research.

RESEARCH MATRIX

QUESTIONS	DENTAL SECOND OPINION	OTHER HEALTH EXPERT'S OPINION	EVIDENCE-BASED RESEARCH FINDINGS	WISE FRIEND'S PERSPECTIVE

If it feels helpful, you can use the table on this page to organise all the information you've collected about different options so you can see an overview at a glance.

ANALYSIS MATRIX

OPTIONS	PROS	CONS
FIRST DENTIST'S ADVICE		
CHOOSE A DIFFERENT PROCEDURE		
DO NOTHING		
DO ONLY ONE PART OF TREATMENT PLAN		
ALTERNATIVE		
ALTERNATIVE		

Step 1 is set up for a relatively straightforward dental decision, such as choosing between a root canal or an extraction for one tooth. In a more complicated situation, you can make, and fill in, separate versions of the research and analysis tables for each of your options. For example:

- If one of your options is a series of procedures such as an extraction followed by a graft followed by an implant, write about each stage separately.
- If you have been recommended a complex treatment plan for issues in multiple teeth, try doing this analysis for each tooth individually.

When you have gathered all the relevant information (which may take some time), move onto the next step: feeling.

Step 2. Feeling

Read back over what you've written about the pros and cons of the options you are considering. Add more notes and highlight the most important points. Then close your eyes and sit quietly with all that information. At this point you may find it helpful to return to the guided visualization from Activity 10.

This activity may bring up feelings and memories of past difficult decisions and/or regrets. Observe and allow any feelings of discomfort, grief, helplessness, frustration or anger (at the dentist! at yourself! at me!).

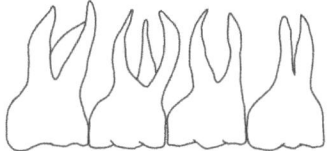

Focus on your breath, slowing it down,
tracking its passage through your body.

Notice where you feel the emotions as physical sensations.

Don't try to stop yourself from feeling bad
by committing to one decision,
or by postponing your choice.

Sit with uncertainty just for now.

If you feel tears welling up,
let them flow.

If you feel anger or frustration as heat in your body,
imagine the heat rising and expanding.

If you feel like you can't sit still for this, shake your arms and legs.

Work with the energy of your emotions using EFT tapping,* Havening Techniques, journaling, dance or other exercise, or by vocalizing (singing/ shouting/ groaning) or other modalities and practices in your personal toolkit to help the feelings move through you without being consumed by them.

Make notes or draw pictures.

When your emotions about the information start to feel less intense, (which may take a while), move onto the next step: deciding.

---

* EFT (Emotional Freedom Technique) or tapping is a simple self help strategy that can help manage emotions, stress and anxiety. Tapping acupuncture points on your hands face and body while you focus on an uncomfortable issue helps some people relieve stress and fears. Look on YouTube for a short introduction to the technique and then you can practice it with the activities in this book.

Step 3. Deciding

If you've emerged from information gathering and feeling steps with new clarity about your dental decision, go ahead and write down that decision below with the current date and time.

But if you feel just as confused as you did before, pick **one** of the options (perhaps the one with the most pros and the least cons) from the information gathering part of this activity. Write it down with the date and time.

Decision-making meditation

Meditate and/or journal on the following prompts **as though you have committed** to the decision you've written down above.

For the following meditation, download the audio recording in the bonus content (link on page 3) or read through the words, and then close your eyes and follow the directions.

After writing down your decision, pause.

Take three slow deep breaths.

Adjust your body into a more comfortable position if necessary.

Then close your eyes and scan your attention the length of your body, from the soles of your feet to the top of your head.

Where do you feel any kind of sensation? What is the sensation? If you could see it, what would it look like?
How could you describe it?

Is the sensation a meaningful metaphor to help you interpret the decision you just wrote down?

Is there anywhere in your body that feels light or heavy? Tight or relaxed? Hot or cold? Expansive or constricted?

Do you feel scared? Sad? Angry? Disappointed? Relieved? Resigned? Happy? Peaceful?

With relaxed curiosity, spend some time focused on the sensations and emotions that this decision brings up.

Do the feelings change as you observe them over time?

Write down your observations.

Checking in with your decision

Wait at least 24 hours, then return to the decision you wrote on the previous page and repeat the decision-making meditation above.

If you feel confident and calm about this decision, start to take action using the previous sections of this workbook to help you overcome any obstacles.

However, if you still feel uncertain or agitated about the decision you recorded, pick another option and repeat the decision-making meditation as though you have committed to it.

Repeat this activity as often as necessary for each of your most realistic options until you feel a calm certainty about your decision.

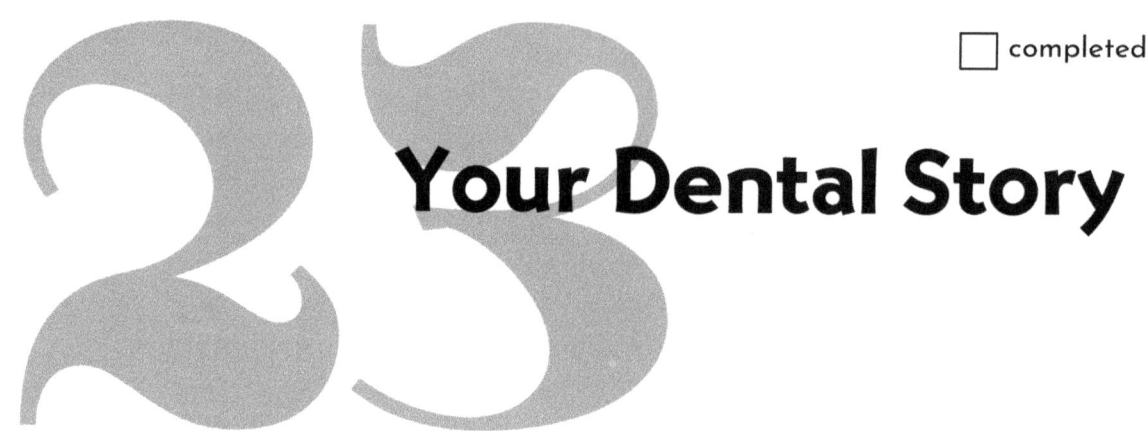

Your Dental Story

☐ completed

In this journaling activity, you can dig deeper into your dental history to work with difficult memories that are consciously or subconsciously affecting your current dental experiences.

This kind of inner work is not necessarily right for everyone's needs and even if it's something you want to do, it may not be your priority in the lead-up to an imminent dental appointment.

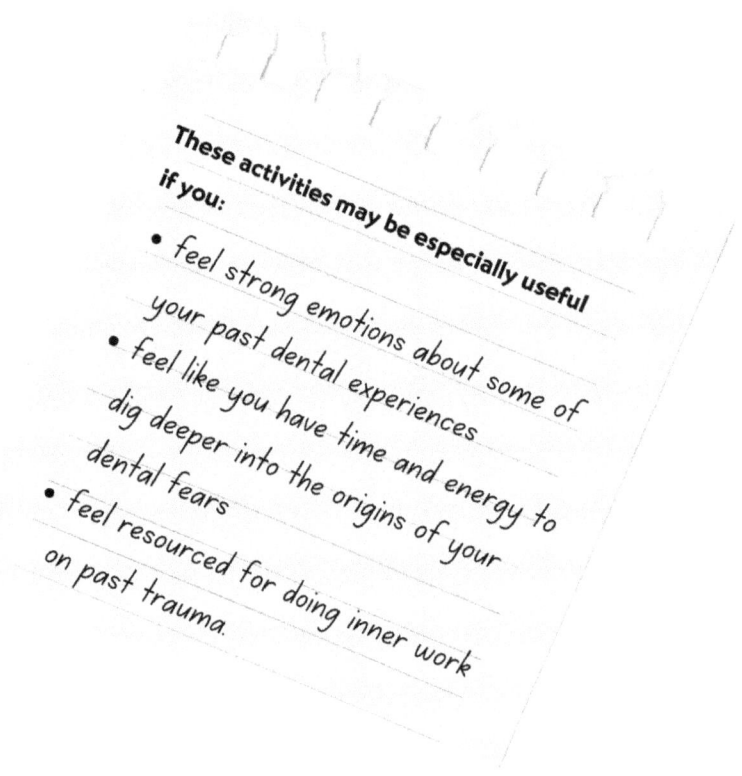

These activities may be especially useful if you:

- feel strong emotions about some of your past dental experiences
- feel like you have time and energy to dig deeper into the origins of your dental fears
- feel resourced for doing inner work on past trauma.

The Murder House (my dental story)

My earliest memory of anything to do with dental care was the Murder House. That's what all the kids called a squat wooden shed that loomed over the concrete playground in between the new entrants' buildings and the big kids' classrooms of Hamilton East Primary School.

Adults called it the school dental clinic, our local branch of New Zealand's School Dental Service, a program that started in 1921 and is still going under a different name. When I was five, school dental clinics were staffed by dental nurses with out-of-date training and second-hand equipment. They didn't have access to X-rays, high-speed drills or curing lights for composite fillings. Amalgam fillings were the norm, and school clinic environments carried dangerously high levels of mercury.

The fearsome reputation of the Murder House was shared in horror stories whispered around the playground. Kids would double down on the terror with an ominous chorus of ghostly noises performed whenever one of us was called out of lessons for a walk to the Murder House. It seemed to be a horrible lottery whether a classmate would return with swollen lips and tear-stained cheeks or reappear apparently unscathed and carrying a tiny white fairy that the dental nurse had fashioned from cotton wadding and dental floss. I coveted one of those fairies but not enough to mitigate my fear of the Murder House.

In the upheaval of our family immigrating from Canada to New Zealand in my preschool years, dental visits had fallen through the cracks. So, my first check-up at the age of five began with a soundtrack of scary noises as I left class to walk alone to the Murder House.

The clinic was cold and as I climbed up into the strange big chair, my bare legs goose bumped and stuck to its slippery vinyl. The dental nurse was a brusque woman wearing a short white uniform, red cardigan and a stiff little cap perched on her 1970s bouffant. Her hands were icy, and her metal instruments lined up sharp and ominous.

As she ordered me to open my mouth to its widest angle, I focused my gaze on a mobile of cotton wool fairies and bees dangling over the chair. I braced myself against the wooden armrests as the nurse began to poke and scratch inside my mouth while scolding me for cavities.

I vividly remember the horrible rumbling grind of the old drill and how it reverberated through my whole body, not to mention the pain. There was no local anaesthetic. Trying to distract myself from the unpleasant noises and discomfort, I concentrated on which fairy I would choose when I had survived this ordeal.

But after a very aggressive polish I was dismissed back to class without even a bee. The nurse had turned away to clean up her instruments and my body was trembling with adrenaline. I summoned up the courage to ask, "Could I please have a cotton wool fairy."

"No," the nurse said, "those are only for good little girls."

Your dental story

I hope that your early memories of dental care are not as brutal as mine!

Unfortunately, too many people of every generation have felt shamed, pained, or overwhelmed at some point in their dental life.

If it feels helpful, use the following journal prompts to unpack your own dental history.

What is your earliest (or most traumatic) memory of getting dental care?

How old were you? Where was it? Who was there with you?

What do you remember about the dental team,
their equipment and what they said?

How did you feel?

What were you told about the dental treatment?

*What did you hear other children or adults
say about going to the dentist?*

What is it about going to the dentist now that reminds you of your childhood experiences?

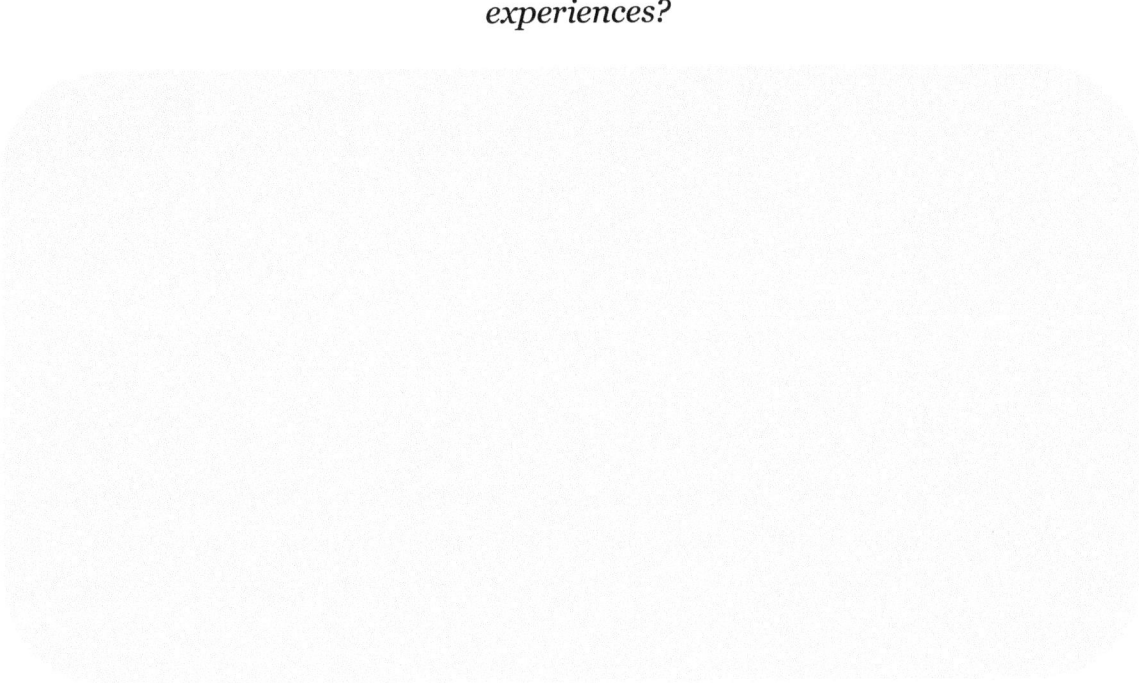

Repeat this journaling exercise with each significant dental memory throughout your life.

When you have finished for the day, close your journaling practice with the re-orienting ritual (Activity 2).

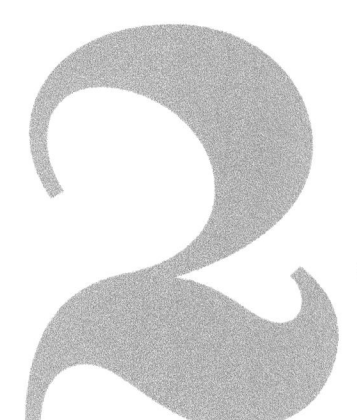

☐ completed

Forgiving The Past

This activity focuses on letting go of the emotional residue of past dental experiences. If you are considering returning to a dentist or hygienist who has previously been dismissive or disrespectful toward you, then it may be more appropriate to try to find a new dentist. But if that's not possible, managing your emotions can help you to improve the existing relationship.

This practice is based on the Ho'oponopono (Hawai'ian Forgiveness Prayer) a traditional practice shared by Nana Veary and other Hawai'ian elders.

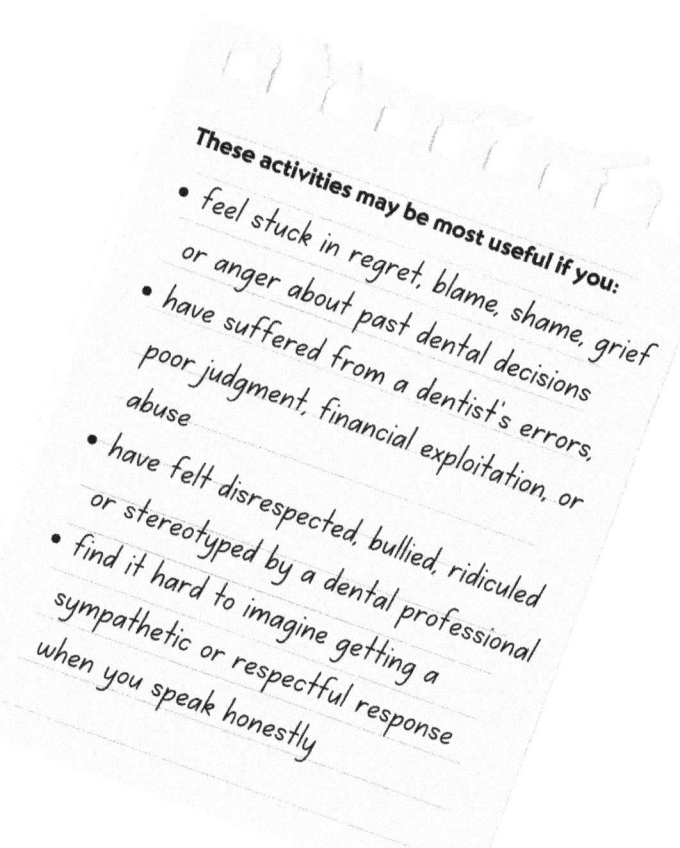

These activities may be most useful if you:

- feel stuck in regret, blame, shame, grief or anger about past dental decisions
- have suffered from a dentist's errors, poor judgment, financial exploitation, or abuse
- have felt disrespected, bullied, ridiculed or stereotyped by a dental professional
- find it hard to imagine getting a sympathetic or respectful response when you speak honestly

Forgiveness Practice

Read through your dental story notes from Activity 23. Pause after each section to sit with the memories and feelings of that particular experience.

Repeat the following words for each person involved in the experience, so that you are addressing them to your dental team, yourself, and anyone else who played a role at that time.

I forgive you.
I love you.
I'm sorry.
Thank you.

As you say this mantra aloud, stroke your fingers together, using the Havening Technique from Activity 13.

Try using EFT tapping or another somatic technique at the same time as the forgiveness prayer.

When you have gone through all your notes from this exercise, close your practice with the reorienting ritual in Activity 2.

25 Dental Diary

It may take more than one dental visit to completely overcome all dental anxiety. This activity encourages you to look for, and celebrate, small improvements over time.

Old neural pathways that get activated with anxiety about the dentist have to be overlaid with new linkages that have neutral, or even positive, associations. This brain retraining process is reinforced with repetition.

This activity may be especially useful if you:

- have a long history of dental difficulties
- continue to feel unwilling or anxious about going to the dentist after trying some of the earlier activities
- only have time or emotional capacity to work through a couple of new activities before each dental appointment.

After each dental visit, make some notes about what was helpful and what wasn't. Before the next visit, review what you've written, and try out or repeat some of the activities in the rest of this book.

Use these pages to keep a record of all your dental visits from now on. Make a few notes soon after each appointment, while the experience is still fresh in your mind.

Date

Dental office/names of practitioners

Purpose of visit

Outcome of visit

Recommendations/treatment plan

Experience in the chair

Date

Dental office/names of practitioners

Purpose of visit

Outcome of visit

Recommendations/treatment plan

Experience in the chair

Date

Dental office/names of practitioners

Purpose of visit

Outcome of visit

Recommendations/treatment plan

Experience in the chair

Date

Dental office/names of practitioners

Purpose of visit

Outcome of visit

Recommendations/treatment plan

Experience in the chair

Date

Dental office/names of practitioners

Purpose of visit

Outcome of visit

Recommendations/treatment plan

Experience in the chair

Date

Dental office/names of practitioners

Purpose of visit

Outcome of visit

Recommendations/treatment plan

Experience in the chair

Date

Dental office/names of practitioners

Purpose of visit

Outcome of visit

Recommendations/treatment plan

Experience in the chair

Date

Dental office/names of practitioners

Purpose of visit

Outcome of visit

Recommendations/treatment plan

Experience in the chair

Next Steps

Thank you for reading and, hopefully, doing this workbook.

If it was helpful for you, please tell others so that more people can overcome dental anxiety in order to get the dental care they need.

I'd love you to tell your dentist about this resource and suggest they make copies available for their patients.

One of the best ways you can help new readers believe that this book could help them too is by writing a reader review, either on Amazon, GoodReads, my website (www.holistictoothfairy.com) or your own social media account.

Acknowledgements

Thanks to all my coaching clients who trusted me to help them overcome dental fears and uncertainties; together we figured out a lot of the tactics shared in this book. I'm especially appreciative to everyone who gave permission for me to share their experiences and advice here. I hope I have done you justice in these pages.

I'm thankful for all the help with fine-tuning and polishing through several iterations from Meghan Wright, Cheralyn Miller, Michal Takacs, Amy Gomez, Daniela Roates, Gill Ramsey, Lynne Durham, Susan Fisch, Chantelle Olssen-Chang, Laura Margetts, Catherine Lee, Sarah Chann, Eleanor Lefever, Morag Egan, and Hilary Tolley. Special thanks to Jessica Gordon for writing the foreword and giving feedback on the draft, and to Elizabeth Rawlings for editing. All the remaining mistakes are down to me.

This book couldn't have happened without encouragement, support or advice from my mentors Andrea Schroeder and Pip Kempthorpe, my assistants Fatin Zainudin and Zoe Taylor, my weekly peer support buddies Michelle Whitehead and Conrad Johnson, and my family, Martha and Louise Simms. Thank you!

Turn the page to an excerpt from

The Secret Lives of Teeth:
Understanding emotional influences
on oral health

by Meliors Simms

Winner of Bronze Medal in the Global Book Awards 2023
(Health Mind and Body Category)

Have you ever wondered whether there's more to oral health than regular brushing and avoiding sugar…

Whether there's an emotional or spiritual meaning to tooth decay or gum recession…

Or why dental problems sometimes rise and fall with stress?

Now you can learn how to interpret the metaphysical messages of your teeth and gum symptoms.

This clear and comprehensive guide teaches you a unique, complementary self-help approach to easing toothaches, enhancing enamel and gum remineralization and getting better results with necessary dental treatments.

Written with empathy and compassion for anyone who has ever worried about their own teeth or gums, *The Secret Lives of Teeth* also has much to offer complementary health practitioners, therapists, and coaches as well as dental professionals.

Natural oral health coach, Meliors Simms, has helped hundreds of people all over the world to achieve better dental outcomes. Now, she unpacks the oral effects of generational trauma, adverse experiences, and adaptive emotional patterns to reveal an effective, complementary approach to oral health.

The Secret Lives of Teeth offers fascinating perspectives including:
- A unique system of Tooth Archetypes to explain **each individual tooth's emotional vulnerabilities**
- Energetic interpretations for **abscesses, bruxism, cavities, gingivitis, tartar, receding gums** and other symptoms
- Metaphysical self-help exercises to help you relieve symptoms **and** feelings of shame and fear about your oral health.

Discover an exciting new way to respond to teeth and gum problems!

Chapter 1. Root Cause

At 3 am the tooth called Rival was throbbing like a siren, intense but diffuse, pounding the front of my head from the inside, but not yet recognizable as a toothache.

My pain slid from ten out of ten down to a nine when I hauled myself up on a bank of pillows. I stumbled to the bathroom for pills, which eventually dulled the pain to a mere six.

Through a thudding fog of agony and exhaustion, I tried to calm my breathing and anxious thoughts. Then I remembered feeling this exact kind of pain before, and the outcome it led to every other time.

Tears started to leak as I pleaded with my body, 'not another root canal'. There was nothing untoward noted in my last dental check-up just a few months earlier, but all my other root canals also came crashing in without warning.

More clarity came with the early morning light, but no peace. The pain started to concentrate into my lower right jaw, confirming its dental origins. At 8 am I started calling around to find a dentist who could see me straight away.

Every one of my six root canals started this way. They also each occurred in, or soon after, a rootless period of my life involving homelessness, immigration or extended travel. However, it was only much later that I saw the overlap between my tooth roots clamoring for attention and my nervous system's inherited preference for flight over fight.

When I was seventeen, an ancestral and personal pattern of running away from trouble served to weaken the energetic roots of an upper incisor bearing the Inner Critic archetype. I had my first root canal after leaving my hometown to escape from anti-Semitic bullying and crushing depression. While hitchhiking and couch surfing, a mysterious onslaught of horrific pain was only relieved by a humiliating dental school root canal procedure.

The experience was a wakeup call to embrace more vigilant oral hygiene and regular dental visits. Nonetheless, almost every check-up for the next three decades resulted in more fillings and every few years another root canal, crown or extraction. Dental interventions usually brought me some respite from pain but did nothing to relieve the feelings of shame, disappointment, and frustration about the state of my teeth.

Through all those years I was consistent with my brushing and flossing habits, conscientious about healthy eating and mostly compliant with the advice I received at my frequent dental check-ups. Yet nothing I did ever seemed to stop the decline. I couldn't understand why there wasn't a correlation between my oral health habits and their results. Dentists subtly, or not so subtly, blamed my supposed bad habits, but I felt that was unjust because I conscientiously followed their advice.

Like most people, I was taught that any problems with my teeth proved I'd failed to comply with the three commandments of mainstream oral health advice, first learned from parents and teachers, absorbed through media and marketing, and reinforced by dentists:

1. Brush and floss daily.

2. Avoid sugary drinks and food.

3. Get regular dental check-ups and cleanings.

In my late twenties, the roots of a left molar carrying the Home archetype were compromised after three years of international travel as a single mother. I was prescribed a root canal for unbearable yet unfocused jaw pain when I landed back in my parents' house almost 15 years after leaving. Unfortunately, the dentist mistakenly removed the healthy nerve of the adjacent molar (Conception archetype) leaving me in pain for another week before I went back to have the procedure repeated.

Within six months, both of those root canals failed and had to be redone by another dentist. A couple of years later they failed again, so I chose to have them extracted rather than go through another expensive attempt to save the teeth. Each surgery felt like a failure, not just of my body, but also of the dental profession.

Underlying influences

Under the harsh lights of a dental clinic, considering emotional, energetic, ancestral, relational and collective influences on oral health may seem ridiculous, even primitive. Like the rest of Western medicine, dentistry has always considered mind and body as separate. Dentists almost always treat their patients' mouths with little reference to the rest of their body, let alone their thoughts and feelings. Mainstream dentistry tends to address oral health in isolation, as an individual responsibility and an individual virtue.

However, my chronic dental troubles came to an end only when I learned that sometimes, for some people, the basic tenets of oral health and dental care aren't enough; that even when you attend to those immediate physical needs, your mouth may continue to present problems. I started to understand that my oral health required a systemic, whole human approach that contextualizes teeth and gums in a web of relationships and environments, both past and present.

The first turning point for my teeth was finding out about the influence of nutrition; not just which foods to avoid, but what nutrients your teeth need to be healthy. Furthermore, teeth and gums interact with complex internal systems that are influenced by your whole physical body, including your posture, your breathing and your gut, what you inhale as well as what you eat and drink, your oral hygiene products and habits.

There are also external influences which can have a more delayed impact on teeth including genetics, prenatal, infant or childhood exposure to drugs or environmental toxins, parasites, malnutrition, disordered eating or mouth piercings, not to mention violent causes of immediate harm to oral health including accidental injuries or dental misadventure.

Yet, I always knew that there's more to me than my physical body. Humans are also made up of thoughts and emotions; we have psyche, soul and spirit. Like all beings, humans have a life force also known as energy, qi, prana, or mauri, which can be experienced as physical sensations and interpreted through thoughts and emotions, but which is itself ineffable (unable to be explained)

Your oral health is influenced by metaphysical factors such as your emotional state now, and in the past, including:

Your family history, your ancestors' traumas, and perhaps even past lives.

Your parents' circumstances and emotions during your gestation, infancy, and childhood.

Your adverse childhood experiences, trauma, or attachment-based hurts.

Your attitudes and your beliefs, where you live, when you've moved, and how you travel.

Your stress levels, your hopes and your aspirations.

What you do every day, the people who talk to you and the people you live with.

What you're angry about and what frustrates you.

Your disappointment and grief, your fear and anxiety.

The secrets that you keep, what you put up with, and what you don't do or say.

Metaphysical influences can make you more vulnerable to physical threats. Physical influences can exacerbate metaphysical factors. The exact combination and timing of the underlying reasons for your teeth and gum issues are unique to you. Understanding the stories behind your symptoms can be just as important for your oral health as any dental or home remedy you can use.

To continue reading go to

www.holistictoothfairy.com/secret-lives-of-teeth